KiDS FiRST
Diabetes Second

tips for parenting a child with
type 1 diabetes

Leighann Calentine
with Robin Porter

SpryPublishing
ideas to life

Spry Publishing LLC
2500 South State Street
Ann Arbor, MI 48104 USA
www.sprypub.com

Printed and bound in the United States.

Library of Congress Cataloging-in-Publication Data on file.

ISBN: 978-1-938170-00-3
eBook ISBN: 978-1-938170-05-8

Disclaimer: Spry Publishing LLC does not assume responsibility for the
contents or opinions expressed herein. Although every precaution is taken
to ensure that information is accurate as of the date of publication,
differences of opinion do exist. The opinions expressed herein are those
of the author and do not necessarily reflect the views of the publisher.
Spry Publishing LLC does not recommend or endorse any specific tests,
physicians, products, procedures, opinions, or other information that
may be contained in this publication. The information contained in this
book is not intended to replace the professional advisement of a patient's
doctor regarding medical information, diagnosis, or treatment.

For my daughter Quinn,
who is a ray of sunshine and whose positive attitude
will take her many places in life.

Contents

Introduction

I'm a parent just like you. I'm not a doctor. Nor am I a nurse, dietician, or nutritionist. But when my daughter was diagnosed with type 1 diabetes a few months shy of her fourth birthday, I had three days to become an expert in all of those fields in order to keep her healthy. We were sent home from the hospital with a heavy bag full of diabetes supplies, a notebook overflowing with instructions and new terminology, and a phone number to call each time we checked her blood sugar or fed her a meal. It was daunting and, quite frankly, the scariest thing I have faced in my life.

If you are looking for a guide on how to manage the medical aspects of your child's type 1 diabetes—how to bring that A1c down a full point in a mere three months or how to figure out the perfect basal rates that keep your child's blood sugar at an even 120 all day and all night long—this is not the right book for you. These aspects of diabetes management continue to be a work in progress for our family. But if you're looking for advice on how to manage your family's life with diabetes; how to streamline the seemingly endless tasks involved with diabetes care each day; how to handle school and sports; and how to help your child with diabetes be a child first and foremost; then pull up a chair, grab a

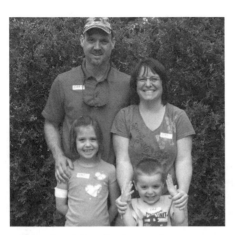

My husband Randy, Quinn, Rowan, and I at a JDRF Family Day event at an amusement park.

mug of sugar-free hot cocoa, and let's chat.

I'll be the first to admit I don't have all the answers. However, I think our family has come to terms with this chronic health condition. We've decided that it is what it is, and we deal with it the best way we can. In fact, that's always my advice: you need to do the best you can with the information and knowledge you have at a particular time.

In this book, I'd like to share with you what has taken us four years to learn. Oh, how I wish that the experienced mom I am *today* had been there in those first weeks and months to give me the tips found in the following pages. What a comfort it would have been to have her put her hand on my shoulder and tell me that I was strong enough to do this. So, let me put *my* hand on *your* shoulder right now and tell you that you, too, can and will do this. You will soon become an expert in your child's care. Before you know it, diabetes will become your new normal, and your child will be happy and healthy. Diabetes will fade into the background and become just another part of daily life ... if you let it.

I can't think of many medical conditions other than type 1 diabetes where the patient, or for young patients the parents, make any number of life-and-death decisions daily. Other medical conditions are overseen by a doctor who prescribes a method of treatment and expects you to follow a very specific protocol. With type 1 diabetes, the care team trains you and then sets you free. And while the nurse educators give you the knowledge to do the basic care—counting carbs, checking blood sugar, and giving insulin—there are so many other aspects to caring for a child with diabetes that these medical professionals just can't teach in a few days of classes. We were lucky enough to be diagnosed at a facility that's strong on education. Some parents get even less instruction than the three-day crash course we received.

That's where this book comes in.

I offer you my perspective as a parent of a child with diabetes who was enrolled in preschool at the time of diagnosis and now attends public elementary school. I won't bore you with medical jargon or indecipherable studies on the latest treatments and outcomes. Rather, I will tell it like it is, hopefully with wit and wisdom, sharing all that I have learned over the past four years.

Things I Know Now That I Wish I Had Known Then

When our daughter Quinn was diagnosed in the spring of 2008 when she was three years old, we were put on a regimen of three injections of short-acting insulin at mealtimes using an insulin pen, plus an injection of long-acting insulin at bedtime using a syringe. Each of these injections also came with a blood sugar check to determine how much of a correction she needed to bring her blood sugar back into the acceptable range. Mealtimes involved counting, weighing, and measuring the food she wanted to eat to determine how large a bolus, or single large dose of insulin, she needed to counteract the number of carbohydrates she consumed.

Mealtimes were incredibly hectic. I felt like the mom in the movie *A Christmas Story*. You know the line that Ralphie delivers about his mom not having a hot meal in 15 years? Yeah, that was me. Add in an almost one-year-old second child, two working parents, and a mostly vegetarian diet ... it was overwhelming!

I quickly learned to automate as much of Quinn's diabetes care as I could. I found we tended to eat the same foods over and over again, so I made a list with those foods, their serving sizes, and their carb counts. Learning about carb factors later on would make counting carbs even easier. Though I relied heavily on packaged foods in the beginning, solely because there was an actual label with the nutritional information right there, I eventually became comfortable cooking from scratch again.

I created a chart dictating how much of a correction she should receive for whatever her blood sugar might be at the time, and a chart showing how much of a bolus she should get for the number of carbs she ate. These charts helped to take some of the calculations out of determining her mealtime injections. They also allowed my husband and her grandparents to give injections without being so nervous.

I decided that I didn't want to reinvent the wheel every day, and you shouldn't have to either. Instead of handing you a block of stone and a chisel and telling you to figure it out for yourself, I'm going to let you in on some of my secrets not only on how to count carbs, which is such a major aspect of daily management, but also on how to navigate school, sports, holidays, birthday parties, camps, and travel while maintaining relationships with your spouse and other children.

The Power of Sharing

Social media has created a whole new world of idea exchange that has benefited me as a parent of a child with diabetes. I began writing a "mommy blog" in 2006 while I was pregnant with my second child, my son Rowan. In blogging years, I'm an old dog! I was one of about 50 moms invited to the *Johnson & Johnson* Camp Baby, perhaps the first large-scale company-sponsored event courting mom bloggers who were becoming big voices in the online world. Meeting the people I had conversed with online reinforced to me that there was value in blogging that reached beyond the computer screen. I met several women with whom I am friends online to this day and whom I see in person at blogging conferences and corporate events. The last session at Camp Baby was a product expo. If I had known then that my daughter would be diagnosed with type 1 diabetes in less than two months, I would have stuffed my swag bag full of the bandages, antibiotic creams, and artificial sweeteners that we now buy in bulk!

When Quinn was diagnosed, I sat on the window seat of her hospital room with my laptop perched on my knees and began writing what I was experiencing. But I struggled with hitting the publish button on that blog post. Should I keep this private? Is it even my story to tell? The emotions were too raw and immediate to disclose publicly. I needed to just stay in "mom mode" and take it one meal at a time.

However, as we settled into a routine and developed a rhythm, I had time to sit back and think. And I decided to write. Months later, I published a post describing the day that my daughter was diagnosed. It was a powerful experience.

I couldn't believe the number of parents who reached out to me with support even though it was not a medical condition they had experienced firsthand. E-mails poured in from parents whose children had been sick and were exhibiting some of the symptoms I had described, asking me if they should see the doctor. (Yes! Rule it out or conversely be thankful that you caught it early.) Readers had a better appreciation for the families they knew who did have a child with type 1 diabetes, and they asked questions about birthday parties and play dates. Soon parents began contacting me when their own children had been diagnosed. These parents sought comfort and advice from another mom who "got it."

In 2010, I launched D-Mom Blog: The Sweet Life with a Diabetic Child (www.dmom.com). I chose the name because many of the parents and patients I was interacting with online used "d-mom" as shorthand for "mom of a child with diabetes." I was finally at a point where I felt like I had the knowledge and confidence to focus on sharing my family's experience. D-Mom Blog quickly became one of the most visible blogs of its kind, and my support group of online parents grew exponentially. Because my blog is devoted almost entirely to diabetes—there actually is more to life than diabetes—my dedication to education, advocacy, and good care for my child has been strengthened.

I have formed valuable bonds over these past few years, and I am thankful to have a core group of friends whom I can bounce questions and ideas off and complain to about diabetes not cooperating on a given day, and who understand where I'm coming from. I have become used to commiserating with other sleep-deprived d-moms and d-dads on Facebook and Twitter at 2:00 AM when we get up to check on our children and can't fall back asleep. With this book, I want to become your 2:00 AM d-mom.

CHAPTER ONE

Diagnosis Day

If you're reading this book, chances are you have already experienced your child's diagnosis day. Since then, your child's life and your family's life have been irrevocably changed. It's a day that you will remember forever, and you have your own story to tell. However, as I've talked with other parents, I have found that sharing stories about this very emotional, life-changing time can be an important part of coming to terms with our new reality. So, that's where I would like to begin.

You Had Me at "Strawberry Shake"

My husband Randy and I met on a chance encounter one evening in 1996. I was out with one of my girlfriends after a shift waitressing, a job that largely financed my education. He walked into the room with one of his high school buddies and, I kid you not, I said to myself, "Now that's a good-looking guy." It turned out that my friend also went to high school with them. Later, I would learn that we grew up about a half mile from each other and attended the same grade, middle, and high schools.

We chatted all evening, and when we went with our friends to a late-night diner, we both ordered the same thing off the menu: a strawberry shake! As they say, the rest is history.

We began dating, meeting for a movie on Wednesday nights, and spending more time together on the weekends. I finished up my bachelor's degree in anthropology the following year. Despite my good grades, the department that granted my degree did not "take their own" for graduate school, so I was forced to apply to schools out of state. A little over a year into our romance I moved to another college town over four hours away. We maintained a long-distance relationship as I finished my graduate degree.

I knew I wanted to marry Randy, but jobs in my field are few and far between. Fortuitously, the archaeology program in my hometown where I had worked as an undergraduate was hiring a full-time field archaeologist, and I got the job. I packed my bags, sublet my apartment, and headed home. Randy proposed to me a week later, and we were married in a garden ceremony amidst lavender irises the following spring.

The Family Plan

Within a few years an opportunity to work in the lab doing research, rather than traveling to do fieldwork, presented itself, and I jumped at the chance. Settling down meant we could start our family, and the planning began. And when I say planning, I mean I *really* planned. I read a book about the healthiest things to do in the 90 days before you conceive; I tracked my ovulation cycle; and when it was time, I knew the optimal moment for conception. It worked like a charm for us.

Nine months later our daughter Quinn was born. She came out ready to take on the world. Everyone commented on how alert she was even at just two days old. I swear she was born talking. By the time the books said she should be able to put two words together, our pediatrician commented that she was already talking in paragraphs. Her early verbal abilities made her a very social creature, and she entertained people everywhere she went with stories and questions.

On the days I worked, her grandmother took care of her. They began going to a weekly playgroup at a local cooperative preschool, and when she was two, she began the preschool program. If you aren't familiar with cooperative preschools, the parents work in the classroom alongside the teachers. You get to know the other children and the children develop relationships with all of the parents. My mother became known to the kids as "Grandma Cynthia" since she more often than not took our family's shifts working in the classroom.

I became pregnant with our second child while Quinn was in the twos class. And yes, he was also planned right down to the day! Our son Rowan was born during the last weeks of the school year, and Quinn was an incredibly proud big sister, showing her photo album documenting his birth and first days to anyone who would look.

Whereas Quinn was a rambunctious almost-three-

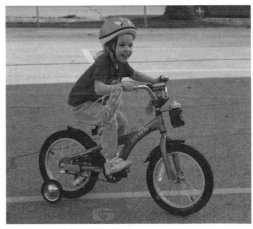

In this photo taken a month before her diagnosis, Quinn was riding her new bike for the first time. She was lively and showing no signs of what was to come.

year-old, Rowan was calm and quiet. He was such a laid-back baby. He could nap in his bassinet in the living room while Quinn loudly, and I mean *loudly*, played. I couldn't believe he could sleep through that ruckus, but he must have had nine months to get used to it while in the womb!

With Quinn, I was a first-time mom who read all the books and fretted about childproofing, the right time to introduce solids, and not washing her clothes in perfumed laundry detergent. With Rowan, I was much more relaxed and go-with-the-flow. I had come into my stride as a mom of young children, able to balance working and home life with the support of my husband and parents.

But it's just about the time you start feeling comfortable that life throws you a curveball and shakes things up.

Something Was Wrong

Spring had finally arrived. The weather was warm, and there was just a month left of preschool. My children were growing like the weeds visible from our picture window, and we began spending more and more time outdoors.

One weekend Quinn developed a fever—a startling 103 degrees. It bounced up and down, responding only briefly to acetaminophen. It was the type of high fever that worries parents, but leaves the nurses unfazed.

I knew she must have been feeling awful because she asked for covers at night. She didn't like to sleep with a cover, and when she did, it was mandatory that her feet be left exposed. Suddenly she wanted to be bundled up from neck to toes.

I insisted on bringing her in to evening pediatrics hours on the third day of the fever. This was a Monday night. The pediatrician, not our own, said it was just a virus and she would likely be fine by Wednesday. Indeed, by Wednesday the fever broke. But then the baby's temperature started to soar. We would endure a good ten days of feverish kids.

On Friday, I was scheduled to work in my daughter's classroom. She needed to get out and blow the dust off. Mounting the stairs to her classroom, parents commented that she had grown three inches in the week she had been out. I agreed she seemed to have grown up and thinned out. The weight loss did not seem alarming at the time.

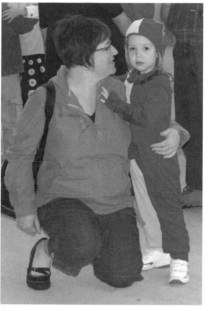

Wearing her clown costume before the circus, Quinn just wasn't herself that night.

I led the class to the music room, and we began to follow the instructor's lead singing, dancing, and tapping sticks together to the beat. I had thought my daughter was well enough to return to school, but during music she was not herself.

"Mommy, I need a drink."

"Mommy, I'm so thirsty."

Tears welled up in her eyes when I told her to wait until the end of music class before she could make yet another trip to the water fountain.

That same night, the circus came to town. She had been looking forward to the circus for weeks. We left the baby with his grandmother, and our threesome headed for the Big Top. She donned the clown costume that had been her only wish the birthday before. She told us that she couldn't wait to try cotton candy for the very first time.

She seemed tired. She felt hot and clammy. She was a different girl.

She did not want to hang from the trapeze bar.

She did not want to jump rope.

She did not want to meet the clowns.

We took our seats as the lights dimmed and the extravaganza began. She took one bite of the eagerly awaited cotton candy, and her eyes welled up. She did not want another taste. She asked if we could leave early. I began gathering our things in darkness, but we managed to prolong the packing until the finale.

We brought our little girl home and tucked her into bed.

Over the weekend she perked up a little. I attributed the episodes of that Friday to the lingering effects of the virus, her fatigue a result of feverish nights, her dehydration and thirst caused by the high temperatures. That night, a mere hour after falling asleep, she awoke asking for milk. Another hour meant a trip to the bathroom. This dance continued night after night.

"Go back to bed."

"But I *need* a drink. I *need* milk. I *need* to go potty."

"You *need* to sleep."

We had a struggle on our hands that we had never had before. Our established bedtime routine no longer existed.

I told my husband that Quinn seemed "off." He thought maybe it was the aftereffects of a persistent virus. Was that wishful thinking on his part? I had an uneasy feeling for about a week, but kept thinking I was being overly cautious.

Something just wasn't right. If I denied her milk or a drink after bedtime, her eyes began to fill with big tears. And then she drank an entire half-gallon of milk in one day. Realizing she had consumed that much milk in 24 hours, in addition to water, I called the nurse. That was a Thursday afternoon.

The doctor said that no child should drink more than 24 ounces of milk in a day. I called my husband to stop by the lab and pick up a urine specimen cup on the way home from work. The next morning I dropped Quinn's sample off at the lab, still none too worried

D-Day

We were scheduled to work at preschool again that morning. It was just chance that we were all at school together that day. My husband had taken the morning off to spend time in the classroom, and since it was also our turn to clean, I left work to go to the school. I figured I would be much more efficient since I knew the cleaning drill. Randy would be able to return to work, and I could drop Quinn at home where grandma was babysitting her brother.

As I began stacking knee-high chairs and tidying up the classroom, my cell phone rang. On the other end was the pediatrician. Not the nurse, but the *doctor*.

"Where are you?"

"At preschool."

"Where is your husband?"

"Actually … here with us."

"Where is the school?"

I didn't like where this was going.

"There was sugar in her urine. I was about to go to lunch, and I was looking over the morning labs. I want you to go to the hospital (literally two blocks away) and get blood work done, and then meet me at my office at one o'clock. Can you do that? It is really important that you do this quickly."

My hands shook as I flipped my phone shut. I told my husband to gather her things. We needed to go *now*.

At the lab counter, I explained that while I realized there were people in front of us, our doctor said this was urgent. "*Please* get us in." The woman checking us in didn't understand one of the orders. It wasn't in the computer.

"*Please*, can you call the doctor, can you call a supervisor, can you ask anyone else? We need to get her in. We are supposed to be at her doctor's office across town by one."

We waited nearly half an hour, eclipsing one o'clock. When we were finally called in, we were met by two technicians and a doctor who came from across the street to perform the test that no one at the desk had heard of.

Quinn's small body was perched on the edge of a large table, legs dangling. The doctor warned us this wasn't going to be easy. I stood next to her, trying to hold her still as he poked her index finger, milking it to fill a pipette drop by drop with her ruby red blood. What took minutes felt like an eternity. He finished and left.

Then, the two lab techs readied their supplies. My husband sat on the bench with our daughter on his lap. He gave her a bear hug to still her as the women drew vial after vial of blood from her small vein. As you can imagine, it was hard for her as a three-year-old to understand why she was being held down and hurt. She cried and cried, and it would take several minutes for her to calm down after the techs finished taking her blood.

Not since the deaths of his parents, one after the other, have I seen my husband cry as he did at that moment. It was heart-wrenching, but we needed to be strong for Quinn and not let her see the fear we were feeling. So, he choked the hot streams back.

We finally made it to the doctor's office. Our daughter sat eating her drive-through grilled cheese and fries while drawing detailed pictures of family members with paper and pens she had found in the doctor's desk drawer.

She needed to go potty, and my husband took her down the hall. I sat in the room alone with the doctor and heard the news: "The glucose level in her urine was over 1,000. In her blood, over 500. She has diabetes."

"Crap."

That's all I could say. I apologized and the doctor shrugged it off.

When they returned, Randy received the news from the doctor, but I don't think either of us really knew what was being said when we heard the diagnosis. It started to hit home when the doctor stated, "You have one hour to pack your bags and hit the road for St. Louis."

The Journey Begins

St. Louis is not just a jaunt down the road for us. It's 180 miles to the edge of the city and takes a little over three hours of drive time. Getting there seemed like an impossible feat.

My car sat abandoned in the preschool parking lot across town. We had all piled into my husband's truck an hour before because I hadn't wanted Quinn to sit alone in the backseat after the trauma of getting her blood drawn.

I had a baby at home, just shy of turning one. I couldn't take him with us. Nothing was packed. My car was not gassed up.

There were but a few singles in my wallet.

We dropped our daughter, just diagnosed with type 1 diabetes, off at our home where Grandma was on her daily shift as nanny, and began scurrying around trying to put plans into action. We are thankful every day that we have a support system that allowed us to leave the baby in good hands, without a second thought.

I quickly packed suitcases with random things for my husband and me. Next, I stuffed Quinn's miniature Tinkerbell suitcase with her beloved Pony, a supply of socks and underpants, a stack of DVDs, and a new player that I had my husband run out and get while I packed *("I don't care how much it costs. This is going to be a long trip!")*. When we finally pulled out of the driveway, it had taken much longer than the hour directed.

Our world was suddenly in upheaval, filled with unknowns. We didn't know how long we would be gone, or where we would stay once we got there. We didn't know what to tell our employers—neither of us returned to work, though we both said we would be back after lunch. But, most of all, we didn't know the gravity of the situation or what was in store for our daughter over the next few days.

On the way, I talked with the nurse in St. Louis who would be expecting us. She cautioned, "If she begins to throw up, she may have ketoacidosis. This is an emergency situation. Do not come to admitting, but go directly to the ER." (We would later learn that diabetic ketoacidosis, DKA, is a serious complication of diabetes that occurs when your body produces high levels of blood acids called ketones. For more on DKA, see chapter 4.)

Until that conversation, I knew that it was serious, but I had not realized it was a life-threatening situation. And we had nearly two hundred miles of striped pavement between us and the care she needed.

When the doctor matter-of-factly rendered the diagnosis in her office earlier that afternoon, I assumed that we would be crossing town and checking into the hospital where both of my children were born. We live in a decent-sized city with a major university and two hospitals. Yet our daughter could not be seen at either one, since there is no pediatric endocrinologist on staff. It was unfathomable that we had to travel so far for her care.

We took the baby's car seat out so that I could sit in the back with Quinn. My job was to keep her entertained while continually assessing her condition. We did not really tell her what was going on. We simply said that she was sick and that we were going to take a trip to St. Louis (exciting for her as we had had a mini-vacation there the year before). I did not think that several hours in a car with a worried child would be fun for anyone, so I decided to downplay it.

We always kept a training potty in the car because you never know when a three-year-old will have to go *right now*. Two symptoms of diabetes, specifically high blood sugar, are extreme thirst and frequent urination. She requested drink after drink in the car, and we pulled over several times to let her go potty roadside. Sometimes we lucked out with a rest area or gas station. We stopped halfway there for a hasty dinner and another potty break.

Darkness was falling as we approached the Gateway to the West. When journeying to St. Louis from Illinois, travelers must choose to go left or right, ultimately converging back on the same road. Every time we come to this fork, we take a gamble on which path is the better choice. We chose to go right.

Ahead, taillights appeared in the dark, and we soon came to a stop behind a long line of cars. We were stuck in traffic high on a bridge above the mighty Mississippi.

And then the unthinkable happened. My daughter started complaining about her tummy. She said her dinner did not feel good to her and she wanted to spit it out.

Please don't throw up, please don't throw up.

I had a stash of Ziplock bags in the car, just in case. I readied one.

"Mama, I don't feel well."

I comforted her with "I know, baby"—a phrase I would repeat a thousand times in the next few days. Stroking her hair I assured her, "We're almost there."

What was I going to do? If she began vomiting I would need to get her to an emergency room immediately. We were sandwiched between hundreds of cars in the middle of a bridge above the Mississippi River. All I could think was that I would have to call 911 and implore them to part traffic for us.

Luckily, she did not vomit, and traffic began moving again.

When you cross the bridge you have several choices as to which way to go. Two different people gave me the same directions: Take I-70 to Kingshighway.

This didn't sound right to us, but we took I-70. It seemed like a good choice because there was minimal traffic. But instantly my husband and I both knew it was not the right way. We began traveling northwest, and we knew the hospital was southwest. As the miles ticked by, I became more and more tense. We eventually came upon Kingshighway and began traveling south.

If you are from St. Louis, you know that sections of Kingshighway, which was our route to the hospital, are a bit seedy. Normally I wouldn't care. But with my sick three-year-old beside me, all I could imagine was that our car would break down or we would blow a tire and wouldn't be able to get help. No businesses were open at that late hour. All the doors and windows were covered in bars, and I had no idea just how far we were from the hospital.

When we finally arrived, I nearly cried with relief. We slowly climbed the circles of the parking garage decorated with cheerful animals denoting the levels and found a spot up high. We carried our daughter, clutching her Pony, to the elevator and across the walkway.

The woman at the admitting desk said they were beginning to wonder where we were. We were ushered to the elevators, flanked by giant fuchsia columns, and taken to the eighth floor. By this time, it was already past Quinn's bedtime, but she would not be able to fall asleep for a few more hours.

The nurse's aide brought small scrubs, adorned with colorful fish, for Quinn to wear. They were much too big, and a hunt ensued to find some that wouldn't slip off her emaciated body. A woman in a white coat holding a clipboard, flanked by two others, came into the room. A dozen questions and a quick exam later and, we were left alone in the room again.

We were told that the nurses would take care of us overnight. They would be in shortly to retrieve us for blood work and begin round-the-clock monitoring and insulin injections to get her blood glucose levels under control. The endocrinologist would see us again in the morning.

My husband left the room, either to forage for a bite for us to eat or retrieve our hastily packed suitcases from the car.

A nurse came for my daughter, and we walked with her down the hall and around the corner to a brightly lit sterile room with a tall white bed. They were going to insert her IV and take blood samples.

I hoisted her onto the high table. Up until this point she had not been scared. Except for the blood draw earlier in the day, nothing had been invasive. But she became frightened as three nurses readied their supplies. I was instructed to hold her down—*really* hold her down. I laid my body across her torso and anchored myself across the bed. My head was next to hers and I told her it would be okay.

She let out a blood-curdling scream, worthy of a slasher movie. All I could do was lie across her holding her still. I could not take away her fright or the pain.

Her screams lasted for the length of the procedure and were so loud that I thought my eardrum had burst. I honestly could not hear anything in that ear for at least 15 minutes. I consoled her as the nurses finished taping her IV in place. Then, the nurses went looking for a midnight snack for our girl—cheese pizza from the cafeteria that is open day and night.

We were finally able to settle in for the night.

While my husband lay precariously on the window seat that doubled as a bed, I climbed into the hospital bed with Quinn to keep her company. She fell asleep watching piped-in Disney sometime after midnight. I wish I could say I slept that night, but I didn't.

The nurses came in every two hours to check her blood glucose level and then returned minutes later with an insulin injection as dosed by the physician. She stirred only briefly each time, worn out from the long day before.

But she tossed in her sleep, rolling in big arcs from front to back and over again. Each time her IV line encircled her and I untangled the web of tubing. Whenever I began to drift off, she would turn again, or it was time for the nurses to prick her finger or give an injection. But it was my job as mother to sacrifice my sleep for her care and comfort.

In the wee hours she sat up in bed, dazed and foggy. A moment later she lay back down. She had urinated in her sleep, something she had not done in almost a year since potty training. The nurses and I changed the sheets and her scrubs while she continued her exhausted slumber.

She awoke in good spirits as she did each morning.

Although her glucose levels had been stabilized overnight, they would continue to fluctuate as the endocrinologist figured out the right concoction of short-acting and long-acting insulin. However, the threat of ketoacidosis, convulsions, or coma had seemed to pass.

We had survived the longest day of our lives and, for a moment, we breathed a sigh of relief. But it was short-lived. We still had no idea what lay ahead of us. What did it really mean to have a child with type 1 diabetes? We were about to find out.

SIGNS AND SYMPTOMS OF TYPE 1 DIABETES

- Higher frequency of urination (including bedwetting in potty-trained children)
- Extreme thirst
- Increased hunger
- Unexplained weight loss
- Irritability or overly emotional reactions
- Fatigue
- Fruity smelling breath
- Sugar in urine (determined by a lab test)
- High blood sugar (determined by finger stick or blood draw)

CHAPTER TWO

Diabetes Boot Camp

While diagnosis day was the longest day of our lives, the day *after* the diagnosis was the most overwhelming! It was time to learn how to manage this medical condition and keep our daughter healthy. Though we had driven 200 miles to get there, we were fortunate to be admitted to a hospital that is strong on education. For three days, a pediatric endocrinologist and the staff—including nurses, a certified diabetes educator (CDE), a dietician, and a social worker—taught us about diabetes and gave us the tools to care for Quinn on our own.

A Crash Course in Diabetes

The hospital stay would include fun and games for our daughter and a college-worthy short course in endocrinology and nutrition for us. While Quinn was painting in the playroom, playing in the rooftop garden, and hanging out at the nurses' station, my husband and I were learning to count carbs, check blood sugar, and give injections. To this day, she has very fond memories of her stay at the hospital, which is a testament to how great the experience can be at a children's hospital.

Unfortunately, I know of other families in our town whose children were so ill—probably in the early stages of diabetic ketoacidosis (DKA)—that they were admitted to the local hospital instead. The staff treated the child until he or she was out of danger, sent them home with a bag of supplies, and told them to make an appointment with a pediatric endocrinologist. I know that, without the intense education we had, these families were even more unsure and scared.

Whether you are treated at a smaller hospital that offers limited education or at a children's hospital with a pediatric endocrinology staff, there are several key concepts that you need to grasp … and quickly! Your elementary knowledge base should include:

- An understanding of what type 1 diabetes is
- How and when to check blood sugar
- What your child's target blood sugar range is
- How much insulin is needed, how to give it, and when
- High blood sugar symptoms and treatments, including what DKA is and how to check for ketones
- Low blood sugar symptoms and treatment, including how to use glucagon
- Sick day management
- Meal planning and counting carbohydrates
- Exercise guidelines
- Managing diabetes at school
- Care guidelines specific to your child's age (toddler, school age, or adolescent)
- Tips to help not only your child but your entire family adjust to this new life

The hospital where you receive care may also provide a resource center with books and videos, spiritual care, social workers, and financial assistance programs. Do not be afraid to ask for help! If you are not receiving the proper education, or are unsure of the information you're receiving, be persistent until you get the answers you need.

Type 1 vs. Type 2

As with most families, the day our daughter was diagnosed was the first time we learned more than just the basics about type 1 diabetes. Our nephew Colton had been diagnosed with type 1 diabetes two years earlier, but since we weren't involved in his daily care, we didn't have much firsthand knowledge other than seeing him check his blood sugar or get an injection at family get-togethers. It's very difficult to get a true understanding of what's involved in diabetes care unless you live with it on a daily basis.

Most people are familiar with type 2 diabetes—they hear commercials for testing blood sugar or they may have a relative who takes oral medicine or maybe even insulin injections—but many people have little or no knowledge about the less-common type 1. Statistics show that only about 5 percent of the 16 million Americans with diabetes have type 1. However, understanding the differences between the two types is very important for parents, caregivers, and anyone else interacting with your child.

While type 2 diabetes is a metabolic disease, type 1 is an autoimmune condition. This means that a person with type 1 diabetes does not produce his or her own insulin and never will again. A person with type 2 diabetes still may produce insulin (although sometimes not enough), but their bodies have a hard time using the insulin properly. Therefore, with diet and exercise change, a person with type 2 diabetes can sometimes improve the body's ability to produce and use insulin, while a person with type 1 cannot.

As parents, we naturally reacted by asking whether we did something to cause the diabetes. It was reassuring to learn that there is nothing you or your child can do to cause or prevent type 1 diabetes. Even medical experts are not sure what exactly triggers the body to develop type 1 diabetes. In the simplest of terms, the cells of the immune system begin to attack the body instead of protecting it. These "T cells" attack the pancreas's beta cells, which produce insulin to help convert food into fuel. As these cells are destroyed, the body begins to lose its ability to process food into fuel. Once this ability is lost, it cannot be reversed. There is only one basic treatment option—replacement insulin therapy.

This can be very confusing for people who are unfamiliar with type 1 diabetes. As a result, you can expect people to think that your child has the same condition as their old Aunt Agnes who has "sugar diabetes." They may offer well-intentioned, but inaccurate, advice. Some common misconceptions include:

- The parents caused it (i.e., they let the child drink too much juice or eat too many sweets).
- The child watches too much TV.
- Only overweight children get diabetes.
- The child will outgrow it or will have type 2 diabetes when they become an adult.
- It's the "bad kind" of diabetes, and they will have complications someday like Aunt Agnes.
- The child should not have desserts and should eat only sugar-free foods.
- The child can't play sports.
- The child won't be able to have a baby when the time comes.

(She may have kidney failure and be found in a coma on the kitchen floor just like Julia Roberts in *Steel Magnolias*.)

* Insulin is a cure.

While these misconceptions can be frustrating and even hurtful, I have found that the best way to handle them is to calmly explain the differences between type 1 and type 2 diabetes. Of course, sometimes it's not worth the effort. There are situations where it may be better to just ignore these comments completely.

You Want Me to Do What?

Once you know what type 1 diabetes is, you need to learn how to manage it. This can be a daunting proposition! I have devoted an entire chapter of this book to day-to-day management (Chapter 4: Diabetes 101). However, before leaving the hospital, it's crucial to become comfortable with the basics, including giving insulin injections.

During our training, the educator showed us the blood glucose meter that we would be using on our daughter and went through the steps involved in checking blood sugar. She had us give it a try on ourselves. I remember the anticipation of pushing the button on the lancing device, not knowing what it would feel like and how much it would hurt when I actually poked myself. My blood sugar was a little low, and I was told that I needed to take care of myself too, including eating regularly.

After we checked our own blood sugar, she demonstrated how to give an injection. The nurse showed us how to insert the syringe into the vial, expel air, and then draw out the liquid, tap air bubbles to the top of the syringe, and push them back into the vial. Our daughter was getting such small doses, sometimes only half a unit at a time, that it was intimidating to look at the syringes with their tiny tick marks. We used a vial of saline and gave each other an injection. This was the first time in my life that I had given someone an injection, and I was glad that I got to practice on Randy before injecting Quinn.

Once we were trained on how to check blood sugar, give injections, and count carbs, the nursing staff left those tasks up to us, of course under their supervision. The goal of the hospital stay is, after all, that you are able to do it on your own once released. There's such an internal struggle when you inflict pain on your young child, even though you know it is necessary to keep the child healthy. Your job as a parent is to protect your children and assure them that you will keep them from harm. It's difficult for a three-year-old to understand that something painful is not only "for her own good," but that you are going to be doing it multiple times a day ... forever.

Quinn barely stirred for the overnight finger checks and injections that first night, but the next day, when she was fully awake, it was another story entirely. Of course she cried and protested, and hearing "I know, I know" wasn't all that comforting to her. However, sometimes all you can do is hold children and let them know you are there for them.

Quinn's memory is that finger checks really hurt in the beginning. She had pristine, tender fingertips back then. They are tough now and marred with tiny holes from years of poking. She says that injections were painful too, particularly the ones given by syringe. She complained for a long time about the bedtime injection. It was given by syringe instead of a pen needle, and the insulin stung, both making the injection hurt.

For me, the worst realization during our education came when the nurse went over severe hypoglycemia, including the possibility of unconsciousness and seizures. I knew Quinn needed insulin to live, but the thought that she could suddenly have extreme low blood sugar that could cause brain damage or death if not treated immediately brought tears to my eyes. It made the life-threatening nature of type 1 diabetes very real for me. The same thing that could keep my daughter alive—insulin—could also kill her. And there we were, tasked with her care.

I know the nurses and doctors tell you that you will get the hang of it and you will learn all you need to know, but it's hard to see the forest for the trees in that moment. Although they probably did tell us then, Randy wishes he had known that, despite the finger checks, injections, and all else that diabetes involves, Quinn could and would have a normal childhood. Diabetes is not a diagnosis that any parents want to receive for their child, but it's also not the end of the world.

Information and Medical Supplies to Go

Since you will no doubt still be in shock and sleep deprived when it comes time to leave the hospital, it's important to have the information organized in a binder for quick reference. You will find yourself referring to it often. You may also receive a bag of supplies. Several of the prescription items we filled at a pharmacy, while other items were given to us by the staff. Our "take-home" bag included:

- Basic information about diabetes management included in the binder used during our training
- List of snack foods
- *The CalorieKing*, a book of nutritional information

- Blood glucose meter, test strips, lancing device, and lancets
- Short-acting insulin, insulin pen, and pen needles
- Long-acting insulin and syringes
- Urine ketone testing strips
- Alcohol swabs and bandages
- Glucagon kit
- Logbook
- Snacks for the drive home
- Phone number to call to speak with the on-call endocrinologist
- A huge stack of artwork that Quinn had produced, as well as a real stethoscope that she talked a nice nurse into giving her

In addition to our supplies, we were sent home with copies of several books that we could read later on as we got the basics down and were ready to learn more. We were given *Understanding Diabetes* and *A First Book for Understanding Diabetes*, both by H. Peter Chase, and *Diabetes Care for Babies, Toddlers, and Preschoolers* by Jean Betschart. *Understanding Diabetes* was a resource I turned to many times to learn more about diabetes management. In the chapter "The Importance of Education in Diabetes," Chase states: "*Families and children need to understand*

> **!** Fill your prescriptions before leaving the hospital so you aren't running around once you get home. If you will be using a chain pharmacy when you return home, see if there is a branch near the hospital. We chose to drive a few blocks to have prescriptions filled at the chain pharmacy rather than use the hospital pharmacy.

as much as possible about diabetes ... [to] help them feel more secure about managing diabetes. It will help them manage problems when no doctor is available. It will also help them minimize hospitalizations for diabetes problems. Families who feel they can manage diabetes confidently maintain control, rather than the diabetes controlling them."

A First Book for Understanding Diabetes is an abbreviated version of the *Understanding Diabetes* book and is a great reference for parents to read in the first weeks after diagnosis. Both books by Chase have a Pink Panther theme. To this day Quinn thinks of the Pink Panther as the mascot for anything diabetes related. She has asked me time and again what insulation has to do with diabetes when she sees a certain home improvement commercial!

Diabetes Care for Babies, Toddlers, and Preschoolers is a quick read that was age appropriate for us, since our daughter was diagnosed at three. It provides much information on caring for the younger child. Both my mother, who babysat my children while I worked, and my daughter's preschool teacher read this book and found it helpful.

What I think you might avoid initially are scare tactics, such as resources telling you that your child's life expectancy may be shortened or that she may suffer long-term complications due to poor management. You can learn more about these things later. Right now, you need to learn how to manage the day-to-day aspects. The reality is that statistics about life expectancy of people with diabetes are based on those who have been living with it for decades. They haven't had the lifelong benefit of today's insulin therapies and technology, so I'm not sure how relevant the data are to children with diabetes today. I have no doubt that my own child's life expectancy will be the same as that of anyone else her age. Not to mention that because we help her maintain a healthy lifestyle, her life expectancy may even be better than some of her peers!

My husband and I have also chosen not to tell our daughter about possible complications caused by poor blood sugar control because we feel that at this age it would be too much of a burden on her and cause her to worry needlessly. She knows that she needs to check her blood sugar and get insulin to stay healthy and that's enough for now. In fact, the Joslin Diabetes Center has studied about 550 people who have been living with type 1 diabetes for 50 years or more. To quote their findings: *"Hyperglycemia is a major cause of diabetic vascular, and neuropathic complications. However, a significant number of diabetic patients, known as the Joslin 50-Year Medalists, remain free from various complications such as nephropathy and proliferative retinopathy after 50 years or more of diabetes."* Just think, these people lived many years with diabetes before the benefit of at-home blood glucose testing, fast-acting insulins, insulin pumps, and continuous glucose monitors, yet they remain complication free. This gives me quite a bit of optimism for my own young child. (For more information about the Joslin 50-Year Medalist Study visit www.joslin.org/50_year_medalist_study.html.).

Going Home

Your child's blood sugar has stabilized, you've learned how to count carbs and figure out insulin dosages, and you've even given a few injections to that poor little protesting child.

Just when you start to feel comfortable performing these duties with the nurse looking on, they send you home. *Wait, can they do that?*

I remember thinking at that moment that my child's life was literally in my hands. She needed constant medical supervision, and, after a scant three days of training, they were sending us home and we were supposed to somehow keep her alive. Leaving the hospital with our child newly diagnosed with diabetes, tightly clutching our binder of information, was incredibly scary.

Looking back, our departure from the hospital was kind of comical. If you thought our trip down there on the day of her diagnosis was chaotic, we had a heck of a time getting back home.

The hospital overlooks a large park, which includes an awesome zoo. Since we had to leave that day, we prodded the staff to let us go as early as possible so we could squeeze in a little fun. We did manage to visit the zoo, ride the carousel, and take a quick ride on the train before it closed. We hopped back on the highway and, when we crossed the state line, we stopped at a Denny's for dinner.

In the hospital, we had a menu that included the carb counts. But did Denny's have nutritional information available? Uh, no. In fact, the waitress was dumbfounded that I would actually need to know the carb counts. So there we were, enjoying our "breakfast for dinner," and I had the logbook, pen and paper, *The CalorieKing*, and various diabetes supplies spread out across the table. I tried my best to figure out how many carbs were in that meal. I called the endocrinologist on duty to tell her Quinn's blood sugar and the number of carbs she had eaten, and to explain my math to make sure I was about to give my daughter the right amount of insulin for the meal. How frustrating!

(In defense of Denny's, they now have laminated nutritional data at their restaurants. Quinn and I have made it a tradition to stop at Denny's to have "breakfast for dinner" every time we make the long trip to see her endocrinologist.)

By the conclusion of dinner, it was getting dark. I don't know if we were overwhelmed or just tired, but we missed our exit and didn't realize until it was too late that we were headed due north on the wrong highway instead of northeast on the right one. Both highways get us home in about the same amount of time, but the highway we inadvertently took has far fewer rest areas, towns, and gas stations.

At about 8:00 PM we pulled over to check Quinn's blood sugar, give her a bedtime snack, and an injection of long-acting insulin. The test showed that her blood sugar was really high. I freaked out and was back on the phone with the on-call endocrinologist. She explained that it was probably a combination of factors, including guessing the carbs at dinner, a long day, and sitting still in the car. I thought to myself, "Seriously? Not five hours into caring for her on our own and I've already messed up?" The endocrinologist told me to give her some fast-acting insulin. She reassured me that everything was okay, and said she'd speak to me again in a few hours when we returned home and checked her blood sugar again.

Could I really do this? Well, I had no choice. I had to gain confidence in myself and my ability to make decisions for her care. Eventually, it would become routine, but, on that day, it was simply overwhelming.

TYPE 1 VERSUS TYPE 2 DIABETES

Type 1 (T1):
- AKA insulin-dependent diabetes mellitus (IDDM)
- Sometimes called juvenile or childhood diabetes
- Most commonly diagnosed in children and young adults
- Occurs when the pancreas doesn't make insulin
- There is no known cause
- There is no cure, and insulin will be needed for life

Type 2 (T2):
- AKA non-insulin dependent diabetes mellitus (NIDDM)
- Commonly called adult-onset diabetes
- Most common type of diabetes in adults over age 40
- Occurs when someone becomes insulin resistant—he or she may still make insulin, but the body just can't use it efficiently
- Inactivity and obesity may contribute to its development, though there is thought to be a genetic influence
- Can sometimes be treated through exercise and diet, with or without medication

CHAPTER THREE

The New Normal

Here we are now, four years after the diagnosis, and we feel like we have a handle on things. Diabetes has become background noise in our daily family life. One of our goals as parents of a child with diabetes is to make her life as normal as possible. Things will be different at first, of course, but as you become more familiar with the everyday tasks of managing diabetes it becomes the new normal. If you had asked me when Quinn was diagnosed if I would become comfortable making decisions regarding her care; if I would become a well-known blogger, mentor, and advocate who travels around the country to learn from and connect with others also affected by diabetes; or if I would say that my child could thrive despite her medical condition, I would have felt too overwhelmed to think beyond the next blood sugar check and injection. But trust me, you get there.

Finding Our Rhythm

While we were in St. Louis, my sister Cari, who already had two years of experience caring for her child with diabetes, put together a care package of some things she knew would be helpful.

She brought Quinn a cute zippered lunchbox to carry her diabetes supplies wherever we went, along with a calculator and a copy of *The CalorieKing* to take with us. She included a small black zippered case, complete with an ice pack that held insulin and syringes. Quinn was thrilled with the cute bandages that her cousin had picked out for her, as well as his favorite sugar-free drink mixes. My sister also lent me a couple of cookbooks that included nutritional information.

It was a blessing to have someone with experience meet us back home with some of her favorite tricks and tools of the trade, even if I was not at a point where I could reach out externally for emotional support. I was in "mom mode" those first few months, just trying to find my footing. Even with someone close by such as I had with my sister, it's often difficult to come up for air in the beginning. I just took it one meal, one blood sugar check, and one task at a time.

To say that life was hectic in those first few weeks is an understatement. Quinn had three birthday parties to attend in the initial two weeks, including her brother's much anticipated monkey-themed first birthday. She had a dance recital in the second week back home, which included two long nights of dress rehearsals and two even longer performance nights. And there were still two weeks left in the school year. Rather than train her preschool teachers right away, I decided to simply stay at school with her since it was only three mornings a week. I took vacation leave off and on until the school year finished out. We also had to train my mother since my daughter would be in her care all day during the summer.

It would have been all too easy to rip our calendar in two and ignore our social commitments. However, by throwing our family right back into preschool, birthday parties, and dance recitals, I was making a statement, both to Quinn and to myself, that life really would go on. I think you need to get right back into the thick of things; otherwise diabetes might get you down. Yes, it requires more planning and thought, but you need to prove to yourself that, yes you really *can* do it.

> **!** Keep your diabetes supply bag packed and in the same place. Having everything ready to go will make getting out of the house much easier. We hang our bag on the pantry doorknob so we can always find it. When we return from school each day, I take a quick glance to see if any supplies need to be refilled.

I have some distinct memories of those first few weeks. Quinn had a field trip to the fire station, and her brother and I came along. We met the class at the station rather than walk the half-mile from school with the other students. We were trying to find the class in the building, and, because I had the baby in the stroller, we kept going up and down the elevators. We went up, and then we saw the class was down. We went back down, only to find that the class was going up. Looking back it was pretty comical, but at the time it just added to the stress factor.

Mid-morning we were in a hallway waiting for the next activity, and it was time to check Quinn's blood sugar and give her a snack. I checked it for the first time in front of her peers and gave her a snack even though the class wouldn't be eating until after the tour. One of her classmates asked his mom why Quinn got to have a snack and no one else did. I didn't have a chance to respond to his question because we were on to the next activity, but since the kids were only three at the time, I probably would have told him that Quinn needs snacks at certain times to keep her healthy and feeling good. Depending on the age of the child, a simple explanation is sometimes best.

At the dance recital we had to check her blood sugar and give her a snack. Even though they were three-year-olds, Quinn's group didn't go on until well past her usual bedtime. This meant that she also had to have an injection of long-acting insulin, which we always gave by syringe. My husband, whom I affectionately call a "stage dad" because he has volunteered at every dance recital so that he can stay with her, had to do all these tasks in the dark! This example reinforces the need to keep supplies stocked and organized so that you can find what you need even in a dark theater.

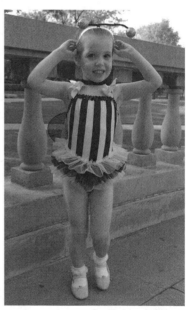

Our daughter missed getting her recital picture taken because they were scheduled while we were in the hospital at diagnosis. So I took photos of her in her bumblebee costume outside the auditorium. She looked so thin, and there were faint bruises visible on her thighs where she had recently received injections. But she was beautiful, smiling, and happy. You would never have guessed that she had been diagnosed with type 1 diabetes less than two weeks before. As they say, the show must go on!

And that's the attitude our

Quinn in her bumblebee costume at her dance recital a week after diagnosis. You can see bruises on her legs from injections. The show must go on!

family has chosen to take. Instead of becoming overwhelmed by the enormity of diabetes and all it entails, we took on diabetes one meal and one blood sugar at a time. Pretty soon the checks, the meals, and the shots blurred together, and each wasn't such a

> Take on diabetes one meal and one blood sugar at a time.

monumental undertaking. Yes, life became more hectic, scheduled, and routinized, but we began to fall into a rhythm, and diabetes faded into the background.

A Bear Named Rufus

I am not saying that it was all sunshine and roses in those first few months. Our child was three years old after all, which presents its own set of challenges. Sometimes her appetite was bigger than expected, so we had to give her injections after a meal. Though she was initially compliant to getting her blood sugar checked and receiving four injections a day, there came a time that summer when she decided that she had had enough, and there was absolutely no way I was going to give her another shot.

For about a week, I had a struggle on my hands. Some days, I had to leave work to give her an injection if she wouldn't let my mom do it. I didn't want to hold her down and force her, but she needed these injections to live. I didn't want her injections to be dramatic and traumatic, but nothing I could say would stop her crying, screaming, and kicking as I came toward her with needle in hand. Luckily, a package arrived in the mail that week that contained the Bag of Hope we had requested from the Juvenile

A TYPICAL DAY

For most parents and caregivers of children with diabetes, having a schedule or routine makes managing tasks easier and can be comforting to young children. It also provides a sense of control, especially in those first few months, when you may feel anything but "in control"! While life doesn't always involve a predictable routine, a typical day for our daughter looks like this:

7:00 AM Quinn wakes up. She checks her blood sugar, eats breakfast, receives insulin, gets dressed, and rushes off to school.

9:30 AM The school nurse checks her blood sugar and calls me if it's high or low.

10:15 AM She eats a snack with the class.

11:45 AM The school nurse meets Quinn in her classroom for her pre-lunch blood sugar check.

11:55 AM She goes to the lunchroom and heads to the front of the line if she's getting a hot lunch. After she eats, the nurse counts the carbs and gives her insulin. Then, it's off to recess.

Diabetes Research Foundation (JDRF). Inside was a little bear named Rufus and a book. I read her the story. I let her check Rufus's blood sugar and give him an injection. And then she let me give her hers. It was serendipity that he arrived right when we needed a way to get past this obstacle, and I'll always be thankful for that.

A bit of advice that we were given by one of

> Give a choice where there is a choice to be given, but not taking care of diabetes is never a choice.

1:00 PM Quinn eats a snack from her snack box on the way to physical education.

3:00 PM The school day ends. She plays on the playground for 15 minutes before heading home. She will check her blood sugar right away if she's feeling low, or will wait until she gets home. She has an afternoon snack.

4:00 PM Quinn checks her blood sugar before gymnastics or dance. She will have a snack on the way, depending on her blood sugar and what time she had her afternoon snack.

6:00 PM We do a blood sugar check before dinner and give a partial bolus of insulin before the meal, following up with more insulin after the meal depending on the number of carbs she eats.

8:00 PM She does a blood sugar check and has a bedtime snack, depending on her number.

10:00 PM We check her blood sugar before heading to bed and decide whether additional overnight checks are needed.

2:00 AM Blood sugar check as needed.

the nurses in the hospital about caring for a young child with diabetes is to give a choice where there is a choice to be given, but that not taking care of diabetes is never a choice. In other words, ask your child which finger he or she would like to use for a blood glucose check. But checking the blood sugar is not a choice, it's a given. Ask them where they would like the injection this time. But getting the injection is not a choice, it's a given. And if a bandage makes a child feel better after a blood sugar check or shot, offer a choice of those, too. Diabetes is a fact of your child's life now. Your child may feel that control has been taken away, so it's important to give children some choices to make them feel like they still have some independence and say-so.

You will learn more about your child's diabetes and become confident in the many decisions you have to make each day about his or her care. Later in the book, I will share some ways I have automated the everyday tasks involved in diabetes management,

SHARING THE DIAGNOSIS

It's natural for friends and family to want to call or stop by in those first weeks after the diagnosis. They only want to help, but you may be too busy trying to figure out how you're going to keep your child healthy to deal with a flurry of visitors. It's okay to ask friends to hold off on visits until you get a handle on things. When you're ready, here are some good ways to share the news and teach people about diabetes:

Young Children

- Read one of the various age-appropriate children's books to your child's class.
- Show the children what's in the "kit" you (or your child) carry so they don't think it's so mysterious.
- Make a collage showing your child measuring a meal, getting their blood sugar checked, receiving an injection, etc., to show to the class.
- Some children think needles are scary. Explain that it's a small needle, not like the vaccinations they get, and that they shouldn't be nervous if they see your child getting an injection.
- Tell them that they will not catch diabetes from your child. Explain simply that her pancreas stopped working and she can't make her own insulin. She has to check her blood sugar and get injections to stay healthy.

Friends and Family

- Invite several people over at once so that you don't have to give the same talk multiple times.

which help take some of the thinking out of it and hopefully reduce time, effort, and stress. Within weeks or months of your child's diagnosis, you will look back and realize that you too are living with a new normal.

- If they are not caregivers of your child, you can teach them the basics, such as the signs of low blood sugar and how to treat it. Let them know that they don't have to make special accommodations, such as stocking up on sugar-free products, and that your child can still be included in celebrations, including eating cake.
- If your child is self-conscious about her diabetes, you may choose to do this without her present.

Caregivers

- Share books covering the basics of diabetes care, such as *Diabetes Care for Babies, Toddlers, and Preschoolers* or *A First Book For Understanding Diabetes*. You want to educate caregivers without overwhelming them with too much information.
- Go over the signs and symptoms of low blood sugar, including treatment using the "rule of 15s" (see chapter 4), how and when to use glucagon, signs and symptoms of high blood sugar, and when to check for ketones.
- Give an introduction to counting carbs and giving insulin if this will be one of their duties when caring for your child.
- Hand out a simple one-to-two-page instruction sheet that includes all the important information at a glance.
- Reassure them that they can do this, too, and that you are only a phone call away if they have questions.

CHAPTER FOUR

Diabetes 101

Managing diabetes requires a parent to wear many hats, including those of a nurse, researcher, nutritionist, and technology expert. In addition, as you master these roles, you must also teach your children how to care for themselves, giving them age-appropriate responsibilities and instilling good habits. At times, this can seem mind-boggling, because while insulin replacement therapy is the only treatment option for type 1 diabetes, there are many tools of the trade. Understanding what those tools are, how to use them, and which ones are best for your child will make diabetes care much easier on everyone.

Checking Blood Sugar

The biggest key to managing your child's diabetes is to closely monitor his or her blood sugar or glucose levels. The blood sugar level at a given meal or time of day gives you information about what they need in terms of insulin and care at that moment. I always gasp when I hear of adults who don't check their blood sugar regularly. How can you possibly know how much or how little insulin your child needs if you don't know what his or her blood sugar is?

Your child's blood sugar should be checked, minimally, four times each day—before each of the three meals and at bedtime. Some children are also checked at snack times and during the night on the advice of that child's endocrinologist and accordingly to the parents' comfort level. Additionally, blood sugar should also be checked any time the child has symptoms of high or low blood sugar or is ill. (See later in this chapter for more information about high and low blood sugar, and chapter 9 for sick day strategies.) Blood sugar levels may be checked before or after physical activity and sports, too. Your doctor will help you develop a testing plan that works best for your child's situation.

Though there are several lines of research underway to develop noninvasive means to measure blood sugar, currently the most accurate way is to apply a drop of blood to a test strip which has been inserted into a blood glucose meter. The meter analyzes the blood, giving a measurement in mg/dl. In countries other than the United States, it might be measured in mmol/L. This number is used to determine what should be done to bring the child's blood sugar into the acceptable range, as outlined by the child's endocrinologist. If a child's blood sugar is lower than the target range, he or she is considered to be *hypo*glycemic and needs fast-acting sugar to come up to the acceptable range. If a child's blood sugar is above the acceptable range, he or she *hyper*glycemic and needs insulin to bring the blood sugar down. As you can see, measuring blood sugar provides critical guidance in managing your child's diabetes. Your doctor will provide you with target ranges and will help you learn how to manage blood sugar levels effectively.

(For more information about target blood sugar ranges, see *Understanding Diabetes* and *ADA Diabetes Care*, both of which are listed in the resources section.)

Lancing Devices and Test Strips

When your child was diagnosed, you probably used the lancing device and lancets that came with the blood glucose meter you were given. That decision is typically based on which test strips your insurance company considered the preferred brand. Well, I'll be the first to tell you that not all lancing devices are created equal. Unfortunately, it took us a while to figure out that there was a better alternative for our child.

For most lancing devices, you pop the end off, insert a lancet removing the protective cap, replace the end of the lancing device, cock it, hold it to your child's finger, and push the button, which sends the sharp object at lightning speed toward your child's once-delicate fingertip. Let me tell you, it hurts. It throbs for minutes. Sure, if I had to do it ten times a day like our children do, I'd be used to it, but it still hurts.

There are several ways to make the experience a little less painful for your child. First, choose a meter and associated test strips that require the smallest drops of blood. When we switched to the Abbott FreeStyle test strips with the butterfly icon, we found that we could lower the depth setting on the lancing device because we needed less blood. Second, lancets come in different gauges, which correspond to the thickness of the sharp end. The larger the number, the thinner the lancet. As you'd expect, thinner lancets hurt less.

Given that people with diabetes can be more prone to infections and neuropathy (a loss of feeling in the extremities), it makes sense to instill in your child a healthy routine for checking blood sugar. Hand-washing is a must because lancing the finger creates a tiny wound that is exposed to dirt and germs if hands are not clean.

Second, a used lancet may be duller, making it more painful, and it may have dirt and germs on it from the last use. I personally feel that lancets are one of the cheaper diabetes supplies, so why not change it each and every time? This is one of those good habits that parents can foster in young children with diabetes.

> **!** Using an alcohol swab to clean the fingertip can be drying, causing fingertips to be tender and blood sugar checks to be more painful. Washing hands with soap and water is milder for sensitive fingertips.

An important milestone in my daughter's age-appropriate self-care came when we switched test strips and changed the lancing device that we used at about the same time. Some parents don't realize that there is absolutely no reason why you can't use a different brand of lancing device and corresponding lancets from the blood glucose meter that you use. We used the lancets that came with the meter given to us at diagnosis, not realizing there was a better alternative for us. I am reluctant to change what seems to be working, but when I saw the Accu-Chek Multiclix lancing device and heard testimonials from several adults with diabetes and parents who used it for their kids, I knew I wanted to try it. What makes the device different is that the Multiclix uses a drum that holds six lancets. You pull off the cap, insert the drum, and it's ready to go. After each use, you twist the end to advance the next fresh lancet. The genius of the device is that there is never a sharp exposed lancet to handle. It is less intimidating for caretakers who may be nervous about accidentally sticking themselves.

Inserting the lancet into a traditional lancing device takes a certain amount of dexterity that younger children might not have.

For Quinn, putting a lancet in wasn't too difficult, but capping the sharp end for disposal was challenging. With the Multiclix, she can easily lance her finger and turn it to the next lancet when she's done. She can also change the drum herself.

Some of the test strips we've tried give errors if the fingertip is touched with the strip. Young children do not always have the dexterity to get the blood right on the end of the strip without touching their fingertips. In our experience, test strips that wick blood from the side of the strip are an easier target and may require less blood.

It was the combination of the two that allowed Quinn to check her own blood sugar at the age of five. Since her diagnosis, someone had always done it for her. One evening I told her to go wash her hands for dinner. Before I knew it, I heard the beep of her meter. She had washed her hands, put in a test strip, lanced her finger, and wicked up the drop of blood ... all on her own. Yes, she had seen it done thousands of times and even talked many a caretaker through the process, but she had not done it all by herself. Now she does all of her own finger checks, unless she is shaky from low blood sugar or is asleep.

I really would like to impress on you that the blood glucose meter and lancing device are not mutually exclusive. In other words, you do not have to use the same brand for each. You should be able to choose the lancing device and lancets that work best for your child's needs regardless of which meter your insurance company prefers. When we switched to the Multiclix lancing device, I saw a price difference in our co-pay of only a few dollars for a supply of 900. It's well worth it to me to pay those few extra dollars for the convenience of not loading a sharp lancet each time.

Continuous Glucose Monitoring

A continuous glucose monitor (CGM or CGMS) is a device consisting of a sensor, which is usually placed on the abdomen, and a monitor, often worn near the waist. Rather than checking glucose in blood as blood glucose meters do, a CGM determines glucose levels in interstitial fluid just under the skin. The sensor takes a reading every ten seconds and the monitor provides an average reading every five minutes. Each sensor can be worn for up to three or six days, depending on the device.

Although a reading is given every five minutes, the CGM must be calibrated several times each day by doing a regular blood glucose test. While this may be a great tool for identifying blood sugar trends, it does not eliminate the need for finger pricks. Any treatments should be given after a check with a blood glucose meter. An advantage of the CGM is that it can be set to give an alarm if blood sugar falls above or below certain thresholds.

While CGMs continue to be discussed for children, they haven't reached a point where they have received widespread use for a number of reasons, including the reluctance of some insurance companies to approve coverage for pediatric patients. I have no doubt that the number of patients using CGMs will increase in the next several years as the technology develops and integration with insulin pumps becomes more common.

If A1cs, basal rates, and insulin-to-carb ratios have you flummoxed, endocrinology offices can provide a diagnostic CGM unit called the iPro, made by Medtronic. This is a "blind CGM," meaning it records glucose levels for several days, but you do not have the monitor to see readings. During this trial, the caregiver also records blood sugar readings from the glucose meter, the number of carbs and what types of foods were consumed, insulin doses given, and the child's activity. The medical staff then looks at the data that they have downloaded from the sensor, comparing it to the manual records kept, and can then make recommendations for changes in care. Insurance companies often approve this diagnostic tool even if regular CGM use is denied. Ask your endocrinologist if you think this might be beneficial for your child.

Multiple Daily Injections

No doubt when your child was diagnosed, you were put on a regimen of multiple daily injections (MDI), including injections of rapid-acting insulin given at mealtimes, plus an injection of long-acting insulin, often given at bedtime.

The rapid- or short-acting insulin is used to correct a high blood sugar and to cover the carbohydrates that are consumed at a meal. This is also called giving a bolus.

The long-acting insulin, also called basal insulin, runs in the background, ideally keeping blood sugar level throughout the day. Many parents are instructed to give this insulin at bedtime instead of at a mealtime so they aren't giving two injections at once. To be most effective, long-lasting insulin needs to be given within 30 minutes of the scheduled time each and every day. We gave this injection at 8:00 PM, give or take a few minutes, and it was accompanied by her bedtime snack.

! Take long-acting insulin out of the refrigerator and allow it to warm up before injecting. Cold long-acting insulin burns, but at room temperature it burns less. If you do need to use insulin right out of the fridge, roll it between your hands to quickly warm it.

Insulin Pens

Injections can be given by either syringe or by pen needle. When we were in the hospital, they first showed us how to draw up insulin in a syringe. After we were comfortable, they asked if we would like to learn how to use an insulin pen. While our hospital roommate's family chose to stick with syringes for both her rapid- and long-acting insulin, we chose to switch to a pen for the short-acting insulin. The insulin pen comprises three parts. The pen is basically a barrel with a cap, similar in shape to a ballpoint pen, but larger. The end is screwed off, and the long, slender vial of insulin is inserted. When ready to give an injection, you put a short, disposable pen needle on the end and you are ready to go.

To give an injection with an insulin pen, you clean the exposed top of the insulin vial with alcohol, attach the needle, turn the dial to two units, and "inject" that insulin into the air to prime it. You then dial the correct dosage and inject. Some patients are instructed to pinch up the injection site, inject holding the needle in place for a count of five to ten, and then turn the needle a half turn before removing it to prevent leakage. (Ask your care team for instructions specific to your child.)

There are many advantages to using insulin pens over syringes, in my opinion. First of all, the pen is not as intimidating in appearance as a syringe. When you publicly pull out a bottle of insulin and draw it up with the syringe, onlookers get wide-eyed. The pen is more discreet because you can quickly pop on a pen needle, prime it, twist the end to dial up the correct amount of insulin, and give the injection. One, two, three, four, done. I think this was a critical aspect of Quinn's lunchtime diabetes care at school because the nurse could quickly give the injection in the lunchroom without having to deal with syringes.

Second, the pens for rapid-acting insulin can measure half units. Small syringes that measure in half units are a little confusing with a gazillion tiny tick marks. Just ask my mother! Since my mother gave Quinn her lunchtime injection each weekday until she went to kindergarten, it was much easier for her to dial up the insulin and inject with the pen than trying to squint at the little marks and attempt to measure the correct amount of insulin in a syringe. Unfortunately, the pens for long-acting insulin do not measure in half units, so we always used syringes for Quinn's bedtime insulin. Some children who are on larger doses of long-acting insulin can use pens.

The Insulin Pump

An alternative to multiple daily injections is the insulin pump. There are several insulin pumps currently on the market, and several others are in development or going through the process of FDA approval. The two basic kinds of insulin pumps are the traditional pump and the patch pump. Traditional pumps consist of the pump itself, which contains the insulin reservoir and has controls to tell the pump what to do, thin tubing, and an insertion set that includes the cannula that is inserted under the skin. Some traditional pumps can be operated with a remote. Patch pumps consist of two parts, including the remote control, which might also double as a blood glucose monitor, and a pumping device, which acts as the insulin reservoir and includes the cannula for subcutaneous insulin delivery.

It is important when choosing an insulin pump to look at all of the models currently on the market. Take advantage of chances to see them in person at product expos and diabetes walks. Request information from company websites, and ask for samples if available.

Some medical practices also have days when representatives from the various companies show off their wares. Be wary of company reps who speak negatively of the competition because they may be more interested in making sales than making sure you make a good decision. Each of the insulin pumps has its pros and cons, but you need to decide which of the features are most important to you as the caregiver and what is in the best interest of your child. Depending on your child's age, you may or may not ask him or her for input.

Choosing an insulin pump was actually a very easy process for us. I requested materials from each of the companies to begin my comparison shopping. I started looking at websites that offered pump accessories, such as shirts and pajamas with little pockets sewn in to hold the pump, and cute pump pouches (fanny packs) to wear the pump at the waist. I also began watching videos of other kids with insulin pumps. For me, seeing a pump in action with a real family and child and hearing their experience is more valuable than a glossy brochure. I saw a video of a toddler wearing a harness to keep his traditional pump on his back where he couldn't fiddle with it. I also saw a pump accidentally dropped in the toilet! The logistics of keeping a tubed pump safe and sound on Quinn's body and the thought of her accidentally ripping the tubing out or it getting kinked didn't feel like an improvement over MDI to me. When I saw a video of blogger Lorraine Sisto's son Caleb jumping into a swimming pool with his pump on, I knew I wanted the Insulet OmniPod for my child, too.

A patch pump represented true freedom in my eyes. I liked that Quinn could bathe or swim without disconnecting, because when you disconnect it means you aren't receiving basal insulin. I also liked that she didn't have to have the Personal Diabetes Manager

(PDM) physically on her person at all times as with traditional pumps. I requested samples from two companies offering patch pumps. The other one wasn't approved for pediatric use, but I wanted to see it. When the sample arrived we placed the OmniPod on Quinn, and she proudly showed it off to everyone who would look. The next morning when she awoke, she told me that she had completely forgotten that she was wearing it while she slept. Knowing that she could forget it was on her was reassurance to me that we should move forward with our decision to get a pump.

Insulin pumps are usually considered durable medical equipment (DME) by insurance companies. Coverage varies from policy to policy. You may have to meet a deductible or pay a large portion out-of-pocket. For traditional insulin pumps, the major cost is up front—the pump itself may be in the $5,000 to $7,000 range. Patch pumps tend to have a smaller up-front cost. Whichever pump you choose, take into consideration the supplies that you will need and their cost.

You might look at these costs and think that pumping is more expensive than injection therapy. It may or may not be. For our family, it costs roughly the same amount of money. There are several supplies that we no longer need, which balances out the costs.

Because insulin pumps are expensive, you need to make the best decision you can at that time. Many insurance companies will not let you change pumps until the warranty is up, which can be five years later. Some pump manufacturers offer a 30-day trial period, during which you can return it for a full refund if you are dissatisfied. Also look for special upgrades for new models of your existing pump and incentive offers to switch companies at a discounted rate. If you choose to go back to injection therapy, or want to take a break from pumping, there usually aren't any problems.

Advantages and Disadvantages of the Insulin Pump

Admittedly, my initial inquiry about the insulin pump was met with skepticism by the nurse practitioner we sometimes saw in place of our regular endocrinologist. She said that Quinn was young and warned of the incredibly increased risk of diabetic ketoacidosis (DKA). I'm not one to take no for an answer, so I did my research, and during our next visit with our endocrinologist I made my case for switching to a pump, resulting in a green light.

Insulin pumping isn't right for every child and every family. It is not a given that everyone with diabetes graduates from injections to a pump, and there is definitely a learning curve as you adapt to the new technology. But that being said, there are many benefits of pumping insulin that are attractive to people dealing with diabetes day in and day out.

- The biggest positive is that each site change lasts approximately three days and replaces 12 to 15 injections. The pump can measure insulin more accurately than you can using syringes or pen needles, giving boluses in dosages as small as 0.05 or 0.1 units, which is an advantage for little ones who require very small boluses.
- Most insulins work best when a bolus is given before the meal so that the peak of the insulin and the peak of the carbs are closely timed. How much Quinn eats at a meal is highly variable. Because of this, with injections we waited until after the meal to give her a single injection to cover all of her carbs. With the insulin pump we are able to correct her blood sugar before the meal and give at least a partial bolus, say for 30 carbs, before she begins eating. With just the push

of a few buttons we can give her additional boluses if more carbs are consumed.

- There are indications that patients may improve blood sugar control by using a pump, and many people have fewer extreme blood sugar swings while on the pump.
- While injection therapy forces a stricter routine of meal and snack times, the pump allows more flexibility in mealtimes. Some families eliminate between-meal snacks or go ahead and give insulin to cover them. And for those who exercise, basal rates can be reduced or suspended to help avoid exercise-induced hypoglycemia.
- One of the biggest bonuses is that it makes diabetes management easier overall. Insulin pumps generally allow you to enter in the blood sugar reading (this can be done automatically for pumps with an integrated meter) and the number of carbs, and the pump calculates the exact bolus needed. The pump takes into consideration the time of day, as well as insulin-to-carb ratios, correction factors, and insulin-on-board (IOB) to determine the units of insulin to be delivered. That's right, no more diabetes math!

Of course there are a couple of trade-offs. With any technology, there is troubleshooting involved. Pump sites might fail, tubing might get kinked, cannulas might come out, and you will have to deal with these issues if and when they occur. Some but not all children have elevated blood sugar in the hours after a site change. Your pump trainer or diabetes educator can give you some tricks to try if this happens to you.

The biggest negative is the increased risk of diabetic ketoacidosis. DKA results from a shortage of insulin; in response the body switches to burning fatty acids and producing acidic ketone bodies that cause symptoms and potentially serious complications. With injection therapy, the long-acting insulin works in the background to keep blood sugar even. But insulin pumps use fast-acting insulin for both mealtime boluses and basal insulin. If you give an injection of long-acting insulin, you know that insulin is working for the next 24 hours. If an insulin pump is not delivering insulin for some reason for a number of hours, blood sugar can rise rather high and ketones can develop. For this reason, endocrinologists suggest checking for ketones any time blood sugar rises above 250 or 300. We were given a "DKA Decision Tree" by our diabetes educator to guide our decision process when blood sugar is this elevated. In over two years of using an insulin pump, I have only had to give Quinn two injections by syringe when I couldn't get her blood sugar to come down with her pump.

Getting an Insulin Pump

I will warn you that getting approval from your insurance company for an insulin pump might mean jumping through quite a few hoops. Some people breeze through the process quickly, but in our case it took months of legwork. The endocrinology practice where we went the first few years didn't typically allow children younger than eight or nine to begin pumping. I'm not sure what their logic was, I know children as young as two who are pumping. I did my research and came to an appointment armed with the reasons that I wanted to begin the process of getting a pump. The endocrinologist told us we could move forward after taking a grueling carb-counting and insulin-calculating test to prove that we had a grasp on the basic concepts of diabetes care. Our insurance

> ! It's easy with an insulin pump to forget all of your insulin-to-carb ratios, correction factors, basal rates, etc., because the pump does the calculations for you. Write down all of your pump settings. If your pump were ever to break, you'll need them to program the new device.

company required a letter of medical necessity and a separate carb-counting class to prove that we also had this basic knowledge.

My husband and I were able to schedule an appointment with a local dietician at the adult endocrinology practice nearby instead of driving 200 miles to the children's hospital. About five minutes into the appointment, it was clear to the dietician that we knew how to count carbs. She jokingly said that I could probably teach a class! We spent the rest of the appointment talking with an on-staff pump trainer who showed us in person all of the available pumps. We found that to be very helpful.

The next step was to do a saline trial. For the saline trial, the pump trainer shows you how to insert the insulin pump, adjust settings, and give insulin. You then use the device for a week, using only saline in the pump. The saline trial week is hard work, in my opinion, because not only are you doing all the things you need to do for injections with insulin, but you have to do double duty with the pump acting as if it is delivering insulin. We were required to keep a detailed logbook showing the blood sugar numbers, carbs consumed, how we calculated boluses, and when we gave them. We

> ! Traveling to a far-off destination? Ask your insulin pump company for a loaner to take with you just in case.

also had to do a site change all on our own. Once the test was over, we mailed back the pump, which stores all the data. The staff downloaded the data and compared it to our records. Finally, the endocrinologist wrote a letter of medical necessity so that our pump could be ordered. Depending on insurance and the endocrinology practice, some children are able to move from the saline trial to begin pumping with insulin right away.

Once we had our very own shiny new pump in hand, we scheduled a pump start appointment with the insulin pump trainer. At this appointment the trainer once again walked us through the steps of inserting a new site and helped us adjust all the settings to reflect Quinn's correction factor, insulin-to-carb ratio, basal rates, target blood sugar, etc. We were up and running.

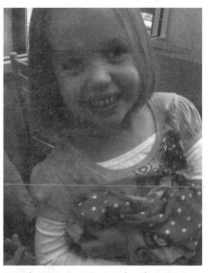

As is our family tradition, the three of us stopped at Denny's to have breakfast for dinner. I gave Quinn her bolus for her meal using the new pump. It was the first time in 18 months that she was able to eat more than five carbs without needing an injection. I asked her how it felt to get

Randy is giving Quinn her last injection before getting her insulin pump.

insulin from her pump instead of from an injection and she said, "It felt like nothing and that is good." In that moment, I knew my five-year-old had regained at least a little freedom.

Ketone Testing (The Best-Kept Secret)

When we were in the hospital after diagnosis, we had to check Quinn's urine for ketones every time she went to the bathroom until we had two ketone tests in a row that came back negative. In the hospital, she could pee into a "hat" inserted onto the toilet. When we came home and needed to check for ketones on sick days or when her blood sugar was above 300, we had her pee into the little plastic potty she had used to potty train. We would then dip the urine ketone strip in and read it.

There are several problems with urine ketone strips. First, I have an axiom that I like to say loudly: *You can lead a child with diabetes to ketone strips, but you can't make her pee.* Seriously, I don't know many young children who can urinate on command. And think of children still in diapers! I have heard of parents who put cotton balls in their child's diaper to try to soak up enough urine to test. I was called into school many days when Quinn's blood sugar was high and the nurse wasn't in the building long enough to wait for her to urinate.

In addition, there is much room for interpretation as to what color shows up on the stick. Do you see those shades of pink and maroon on the side of the ketone test strips bottle? It's not always easy to discern if ketones are negative, trace, moderate, or large based on the color.

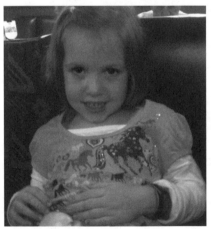

One of the biggest negatives I see to using urine ketone strips is that they lag behind by about two hours. Ketones in the urine have actually been filtered by the kidneys; therefore, a urine ketone test gives you a picture of what was going on in your child's body about two hours prior. The stick could show that your child is negative for ketones when, in fact, they could be building up.

Quinn is having her first meal in a year and a half without having an injection because of her new pump.

I think one of the best-kept secrets in diabetes management of younger children is the blood ketone meter. Unfortunately, I didn't find out about it until the middle of Quinn's kindergarten year. I now sing its praises and highly recommend using a blood ketone meter over urine ketone test strips.

The process of using a blood ketone meter is similar to checking blood sugar. You lance the finger and apply blood to a special test strip. In a few seconds, the meter gives you an actual number, so there is no guessing whether it is negative, trace, moderate, or large. Where the urine test lags behind by two hours, the blood ketone test gives real-time results. It lets you know if there are ketones floating around your child's system *right now*, allowing you to quickly treat. And the best part is that any caregiver who can check blood sugar can also check blood ketones. It is also easy to check children for ketones in the night without waking them.

The downsides to blood ketone strips are that they are expensive and that they expire relatively soon, usually within one to two years of purchase. Urine ketone strips are cheap. Blood ketone strips cost about $5 each before insurance coverage, and some policies don't cover them. Our co-pay for blood ketone strips brings their cost well below the $5 per strip, and, for us, the convenience makes the price worth it. If your insurance company says that they do not cover blood ketone strips, you can ask your doctor to write a letter of medical necessity indicating that it is a more accurate and accessible way for you to assess your child's blood ketone level. Additionally, you can ask your insurance company for an override.

Hypoglycemia (Low Blood Sugar)

Hypoglycemia occurs when the level of sugar in the blood falls below a certain threshold, and the body doesn't have enough glucose to use for fuel. While it has many causes, ranging from a missed meal, exercising, a mistaken insulin dosage, or insulin given to cover a meal peaking before the carbs do, treatment involves strategies to raise blood sugar levels.

Each child with diabetes may experience low blood sugar differently and may use varying words to describe it. When Quinn was younger, she would often complain that she was *really* hungry. As she got older, she began saying that she felt shaky, that her legs were wobbly or wouldn't work, or that she felt like she was going to "flop over." It's important to pay attention to your child's particular symptoms and how he or she expresses them so you can be on the lookout for those symptoms. When Quinn was younger, I always told teachers that if she said she was very hungry, her blood sugar needed to be tested right away.

Your diabetes educator will teach you how to handle blood sugar lows. You'll learn to determine if the hypoglycemia is mild, moderate, or severe, and how to react in each situation.

> ❗ Hypoglycemia can also be delayed, occurring eight to 12 hours after physical activity. For instance, if Quinn has an afternoon or evening exercise class, her blood sugar sometimes dips around 2:00 AM.

Mild Hypoglycemia and the Rule of 15s

For mild hypoglycemia, the "rule of 15s" can generally be followed and repeated until blood sugar rises to acceptable levels. The premise is to give 15 grams of carbs or fast-acting sugar, wait 15 minutes to allow the sugar to begin working, and retest, repeating with 15 grams of carbs every 15 minutes until the blood sugar is back in range. However, your doctor will help you figure out what

is best for your child. The important thing is to test, treat, test, and
repeat until the child is no longer
hypoglycemic.

Fast-acting carbs include:

! Open jars of glucose tablets and caps of cake icing gel ahead of time. Shaky hands might not be able to unwrap the safety seal on jars, and some tubes of gel require scissors to open.

- 4 oz. (1/2 cup) juice, which is the size of a small juice box
- 3 to 4 glucose tablets, which have 4 carbs each
- 3 to 4 tsp of table sugar, each teaspoon is 4 g carbs
- 4 oz. (1/2 cup) of regular soda
- 10 to 15 Skittles; each Skittle is 1 g carb
- 2 rolls of Smarties; each roll is 6 g carbs

If it will be more than an hour until the next scheduled snack or meal, an additional snack including carbs and protein may be given to keep blood sugar stable. Carb plus protein snacks include small protein bars, 1 cup of milk, a cheese or peanut butter sandwich, and 3 to 6 crackers with cheese or peanut butter. Chocolates are not usually recommended for treating low blood sugar because the fat content makes them slower to absorb.

Moderate Hypoglycemia

During moderate hypoglycemia, a child may be groggy, confused, very shaky, or just out of it. Choking is a concern. If a child is low and groggy, glucose gel or cake icing gel can be massaged into the cheek, and the treatment for the low continued, following the rule of 15s. Solid forms of fast-acting sugar can be given once the child

! Don't throw away that stash of holiday candy. Smarties, Skittles, Swedish Fish, and other sugary candies can be used to treat low blood sugar. Eating candy for low blood sugar is an unexpected perk of having diabetes!

is more alert and blood sugar levels begin to come up.

Severe Hypoglycemia

I think the biggest fear parents have is that their child will have a severe hypoglycemic event. If a child is unconscious or is having a seizure, a glucagon injection must be given *immediately*, and 911 needs to be called.

A glucagon emergency kit consists of a vial containing glucagon in a tablet or powder form and a syringe, which contains a liquid diluting solution. These two components are housed in a hard red or orange rectangular plastic box. The kit will contain instructions for administering the glucagon. Be sure to read the instructions ahead of time so that you know what to do when you may need to use the kit. Your endocrinologist will give you the appropriate dosage for your child and tell you how to adjust the next dosage of insulin if needed.

> ! Keep glucagon in the same location so that everyone knows where it is in case of an emergency.

After administering glucagon, check the blood sugar again in ten minutes. If the child is still unconscious and the blood sugar is still low, the dose can be repeated. If the child regains consciousness, she can have sips of juice, soda, or sugar water, followed by a snack with protein.

Ask your medical team if they prefer that 911 be called immediately if the child is unconscious or seizing, or if they want you to give an initial injection of glucagon to see if the child regains consciousness and her blood sugar rises. I instruct our caregivers and school staff to auto-

> ! Save expired glucagon kits to use as practice. Familiarize yourself with the steps involved and practice injecting into an orange. Expired kits can be used to train school staff and caregivers.

NEVER LEAVE HOME WITHOUT IT!

There are several items that your child should always have when leaving the house. No matter the type of insulin therapy, your child should always carry a supply pouch with a blood glucose meter (and accompanying test strips, lancing device, and lancets) and a source of fast-acting sugar such as glucose tablets or juice. They should also wear a medical ID bracelet or necklace, that at least says "diabetic." I prefer an engraved tag that states my child's name, says that she has diabetes and an insulin pump, and gives both mine and my husband's cell phone numbers. In an emergency, police, firefighters, and EMTs need to identify your child's medical condition quickly to give the appropriate medical care.

matically call 911, since they are not as comfortable in the care of my child, and I take the "better safe than sorry" approach.

Treating Lows at Night

During the nighttime, you may worry about your child developing cavities from the sugary low blood sugar treatments. Juice is my go-to hypoglycemia treatment during the night because Quinn can drink it without really waking up, and the straw takes the sugary liquid past her teeth. I also try to remember to have her take a drink of water after she has juice to cleanse her mouth. We've chosen not to make Quinn brush her teeth during the night if she's received sugary treatments. However, I've decided against candy as an overnight low treatment because it is sticky and more likely to cause cavities. And while I do keep glucose tablets in our overnight kit upstairs, Quinn has a difficult time chewing and swallowing when she's half asleep. If she is low during the night, I like to follow up with a glass of milk, because of the protein, and I may reduce her basal rate on her insulin pump depending on the time of night.

Hyperglycemia (High Blood Sugar)

Hyperglycemia, or high blood sugar, occurs when blood sugar is elevated above the normal range as set by your endocrinologist. Causes of high blood sugar include: eating food without the proper amount of corresponding insulin; eating high-sugar-content foods that aren't matched by the insulin; hormones such as growth hormone, glucagon, and adrenaline; steroids, which are sometimes prescribed for other medical conditions; illness; growth spurts; menstruation; and anger. The condition can also occur as a rebound after treating low blood sugar. High blood sugar can result from bad insulin. And for those using an insulin pump, pump failures such as a bubble or kink in the tubing, an empty insulin reservoir, a bent cannula or cannula that has come out, or a leak in the infusion set can cause a high.

Some symptoms of high blood sugar include lethargy, an overall crummy feeling, extreme thirst, and frequent urination. Your child may have had these symptoms at diagnosis. For Quinn, both at diagnosis and to this day, emotional swings are a symptom. If her blood sugar is very high, she is easily upset and cries quickly. Some children experience aggressive behavior or behavior that is not normal for them.

I remember that during Quinn's kindergarten year I met her on the school steps and saw her head hung low. She told me she was so bad that day that the teacher had to write a note home. It seems that Quinn lashed out several times, including throwing a toy and shoving a boy. I had a long talk with her about her behavior. Later that night, as I logged her numbers from the day, I noticed they were all in the very high 200's. The teacher and I discussed how, while Quinn needs to be held accountable for her actions, her blood sugar had been high all day, which can make her volatile. She hasn't had a day at school like that since.

The obvious treatment for high blood sugar is to give a correction of insulin. Your child may need extra fluids and lots of trips to the bathroom until the blood sugar comes back down. For blood sugar above 250 or 300, as suggested by your endocrinologist, ketones should be checked. If the child uses an insulin pump, you should troubleshoot to see if the issue is with the pump.

! Is your child's blood sugar unexpectedly above 300?

● Have your child wash his or her hands thoroughly and check that blood sugar again. Sugary residue on fingertips can be detected by test strips, resulting in inaccurate readings. Double check really high blood sugar before giving large corrections ... just in case.

If a high blood sugar is a single occurrence, it might be chalked up to a missed bolus, incorrect carb counting, or a high-carb or sugary meal. I know there are certain foods that make Quinn's blood sugar spike high, and I have to develop a strategy to deal with them either preemptively or after the fact. But if you see a pattern emerging, it might be time to look at insulin-to-carb ratios and/or basal rates. I always reread relevant sections of *Think Like a Pancreas*, written by Gary Scheiner, when I'm dealing with carb-ratio and basal-rate issues. I also fax my blood sugar logs to the diabetes educator to discuss possible causes and changes.

Just recently, we had a weekend when I couldn't keep Quinn's blood sugar in range, and she spent three days in the low 200s. Correction after correction didn't bring her down. Opening a fresh bottle of insulin didn't work. I was at my wit's end thinking we needed a complete overhaul of her basal rates or that the high blood sugar readings were an indication of oncoming illness. After we discussed it with our diabetes educator, her blood sugar returned to normal, and we decided that the spike was related to her recent growth spurt.

(For more information on illness and high blood sugar, see chapter 9.)

CHAPTER FIVE

Diabetes Central

In the last chapter, we discussed the basics of diabetes care—monitoring blood sugar, delivering insulin, and dealing with low and high blood sugar. In this chapter, I'd like to give you a few "tricks of the trade" that I've found make managing diabetes easier.

In the beginning, I think one of the most surprising things about Quinn's care was the amount of "stuff" that was required and the amount of trash that was generated. The necessary supplies can easily take over your house, your car, and an entire cabinet, if you let it. I believe good organization is the key to making diabetes management less stressful. Having things when you need them, where you need them reduces the amount of time it takes to do the tasks associated with your child's care.

The Supply Cabinet

I have several strategies for keeping supplies organized and at hand. In our old house, we were tight on space. I kept large quantities of supplies in a file box in the hall closet. I also had a shoe-sized plastic storage box where I kept one to two boxes of everything we used so that I could refill our small supply kit, which we kept on the counter. I purchased the small supply kit at a craft store, which was designed to hold embroidery floss. It had adjustable compartments that I could fit to the size I needed.

There are so many items that we use over and over, some four times a day or more—the glucose monitor, calculator, ketone strips, pen needles, bandages, antibiotic ointment, syringes, test strips, lancets, and alcohol swabs. This box, along with our Novolog Jr. insulin pen, logbook, notebook, and the book *The CalorieKing*, sat on the kitchen counter.

When we moved to our new house, one of the very first tasks was designating a diabetes supply cabinet and drawer. In the cabinet, I keep boxes of insulin pump supplies, test strips, lancets, blood ketone strips, alcohol swabs, syringes, and jars of glucose tablets. For most of these items, I fill our prescriptions for a 90-day supply. When new supplies come into the house, I take a few minutes to organize the cabinet, making sure that items with the nearest expiration are at the front so they can be used first.

The drawer beneath this cabinet holds the small supply kit I described above. It also holds nutrition brochures from restaurants, *The CalorieKing*, calculator, alcohol swabs, cotton swabs, bandages, waterproof tape, a glucagon kit, refillable travel-size glucose tablet containers, and other small items.

Insulin Storage

Long-term storage of insulin should be in the refrigerator. However, an open vial of insulin can be kept at room temperature and used generally within 28 to 30 days. Read the documentation that comes with your particular insulin for storage temperatures and times, but generally open vials of insulin can be kept at room temperature as long as extreme heat and cold are avoided. In other words, don't leave your child's supply bag in your car on a hot summer day. Cold insulin burns when injected. When using a bottle of insulin straight from the fridge, roll it between your hands to warm it up first.

If you are concerned about heat, you can carry insulin on the go by using an insulated bag or pouch. You can even use an ice pack, though you don't want to put insulin directly on ice. When we travel in the summer, I put the insulin in a small plastic container and then place it at the top of our cooler. There is a product on the market, called the Frio cooling wallet, which will keep insulin cold for several days. This is an ideal solution for families who travel or camp. To use the Frio cooling wallet, you submerge it in cold water, which activates crystals inside, turning them into a gel. According to the Frio website (www.frioinsulincoolingcase.com), it will keep insulin cool for a minimum of 45 hours, even in 100-degree weather. It can also insulate insulin from freezing. The Frio wallet can be used again and again.

Diabetes Preparedness Kit

Quinn learned about "preparedness" at school and had the idea to make a diabetes preparedness kit at home. Every part of the country has some type of severe weather, and you need to be prepared in case you have to take shelter or leave the house quickly. I'm not sure why I hadn't thought of this before. In the past when we heard tornado sirens, I swooped up some supplies and ran downstairs. Now we have a kit stocked with everything we might need (except insulin), and I keep it in the pantry where we take cover. We store insulin in the refrigerator because it needs to be kept cool, but we can quickly grab it if needed.

Keep your kit in a designated spot so that it can be grabbed quickly, and don't forget to rotate any supplies that might expire. The plastic container we purchased has two interlocking tiers. The diabetes supplies are in the top tier, and bottled water and snacks are in the bottom. Because this kit is stocked with everything we need, we also take the kit with us when we travel or go camping, or when Quinn has a sleepover at her grandparents' house.

Saving Money

You have a long list of supplies that you need to stock in that cabinet and in your preparedness kit, but

DIABETES PREPAREDNESS KIT

(Tailor to the supplies that you use.)
- Plastic container, ideally with a handle so that it's portable
- Blood glucose meter
- Blood glucose test strips
- Blood ketone meter and blood ketone strips OR urine ketone strips
- Lancing device
- Lancets
- Alcohol swabs
- Syringes (for both MDI and pump users)
- Insulin pen (if you use it)
- Pen needles (if you use them)
- Insulin pump supplies (enough for two changes)
- Glucose tablets or other quick acting source of sugar
- Cake icing gel
- Glucagon kit
- Small scissors
- Waterproof tape (if you use it)
- Baby oil or adhesive remover
- First aid kit
- Frio cooling wallet
- Flashlight
- Bottled water
- Protein bars and other snacks

how do you pay for it all? I have a few strategies for savings that can really add up.

Visit the websites of the makers of the diabetes supplies you use to look for coupons and to sign up for e-mail lists to receive notifications. I recently saw a coupon from an insulin maker that allowed patients to fill their prescription for free for six months. Free!

Many of the companies offer savings cards that can be presented to the pharmacist and used on top of your private insurance benefit. For example, the savings program for the test strips we use will pay up to $50 a month on our test strips after I pay $15 out-of-pocket. My co-pay through my insurance company is $65, the savings card pays $50, and all I pay is $15. Some companies offering savings cards also provide free meter batteries and control solution if you call and ask for them. Additionally, many companies have patient assistance programs, which are often based on income level or are granted to patients without private insurance.

Ask your pharmacist and your insurance company for the co-pay amount if a prescription is filled for a 30-day supply versus a 90-day supply. Often a 90-day supply comes with a savings, but not always.

If you have a deductible on your insurance plan and you have met the out-of-pocket maximum for the year, make sure to fill any supplies that fall under this coverage. Often insulin pump and continuous glucose monitor supplies fall under durable medical equipment, not the pharmacy benefit, and can be included in the out-of-pocket expenses. Find out if your insurance plan year ends on December 31st or June 30th, and max out your benefits before the new plan year begins and new deductibles must be met.

If you and your spouse are both employed, ask about covering family members on both policies if possible. Often one policy will pick up where the other leaves off, and savings may exceed any additional premiums.

And finally, take advantage of Flexible Spending Accounts (FSAs) through employers. Employees can designate a dollar amount to come out of each paycheck to go into their accounts. This designated money is not taxed. Typically the money for the entire year is available from day one, which is great if you are making a costly purchase such as an insulin pump. Some FSAs provide a debit card which can be used at pharmacies and will deduct the cost of prescriptions and doctor visits directly from the account. For some items, you are reimbursed after providing documentation. Some over-the-counter items such as glucose tablets can even be purchased with the FSA account, but recent regulations require a prescription for these normally nonprescription items stating that they are medically necessary. Check with your FSA administrator for guidelines. Beware that you need to use or lose the money you put into an FSA; don't put in more money than you think your family will realistically use during the plan year.

What to Do With All That Garbage

Four or more injections and a half dozen or more blood sugar checks each and every day creates a lot of garbage. Unfortunately, you can't just toss it in the trash. So how do you safely dispose of all of the "stuff"? Well, there might not be a good answer.

Sharps including syringes, pen needles, and lancets need to be properly disposed of so that you don't put anyone at risk of injury or infection. Some states have specific laws regarding storage and disposal of sharps. Check with your local hospital, pharmacy, or public health district to see if there are any sharps collection programs in your area. Until recently, our local hospital provided free sharps containers, which they also collected and disposed of properly.

If there is no specific law in your state and no collection program, sharps containers can be purchased at pharmacies, though they are often small and expensive. An alternative is to use an empty detergent bottle. Fill the bottle leaving room at the top, since an overly full container is more likely to get punctured. Tape the cap shut, and use permanent marker to label the bottle with "sharps." In many areas it is acceptable to put this into the regular household trash. I personally feel that local government agencies and hospitals have a responsibility to provide low- or no-cost sharps disposal programs rather than let sharps go into landfills, but unfortunately many of us are left no option but to fill detergent bottles and put them out with the trash.

Visit these websites for more information about safe handling and disposal of sharps, including information by state:

- Environmental Protection Agency
  www.epa.gov/osw/nonhaz/industrial/medical/disposal.htm
- Coalition for Safe Community Needle Disposal
  www.safeneedledisposal.org/
- U.S. Food and Drug Administration
  www.fda.gov/MedicalDevices/ProductsandMedical
  Procedures/HomeHealthandConsumer/Consumer
  Products/Sharps/ucm20025647.htm

CHAPTER SIX

Let Them Eat Cake

Much of diabetes management revolves around food—making appropriate choices and counting carbs. This might seem daunting at first, and it definitely adds to meal prep times, but there are several ways to streamline the process. The diabetes "diet" is really the healthy diet that everyone ought to strive for; but it should also include treats, within reason, to allow your child to share in celebrations and not be differentiated from his or her peers.

Working with a Dietician

When our daughter was diagnosed with diabetes, a large portion of our initial education was with a dietician. Working with a dietician can be valuable for not only families who are new to diabetes management, but also for those who feel like they are in a rut, serving the same foods over and over. If you don't feel confident making good food choices or counting carbs, a dietician can provide helpful guidance.

My Philosophy on Food

Here's my philosophy when it comes to food—everything in moderation. Almost every aspect of diabetes management is

A DIETICIAN ON YOUR TEAM

Courtney Slater, RD, LD

Dietitians can be a great addition to your or your child's diabetes care team. However, when searching for a dietitian or diabetes educator, be sure to look for someone with the proper credentials—someone who has RD (Registered Dietitian) beside her or his name. This means he or she has completed the necessary schooling and has successfully passed the credentialing exam for dietetics. Most states also require licensing in order to practice nutrition—you may also see the letters LD or LDN behind the educator's name. Be wary of anyone touting themselves as a "nutritionist" but without the letters "RD" after his or her name. The word "nutritionist" is not a regulated term and can be used by anyone claiming to be an "expert." The dietitian should also have a registration certificate visible in her or his office. If you don't notice it, ask to see it. It's important to make sure you're getting your care from an expert in the field of nutrition.

Growing up with diabetes, I saw quite a few dietitians in my day. Some methods of teaching worked wonders for my diabetes care, while others rendered me less than enthusiastic about diabetes management. With these personal experiences added to my bag of "dos and don'ts," I became a dietitian. Having the unique experience of being a dietitian, while also living life with diabetes, I dove headfirst into diabetes education. Even though I work as a diabetes educator now, I still occasionally make appointments with dietitians and certified diabetes educators to help keep me on track. Sometimes a different point of view, or talking out my troubles with someone else, is what I need to help guide me on my diabetes journey.

My patients who come for diabetes education are lucky they have a dietitian who has "been there, done that" in terms of living with diabetes. While that experience isn't always available, there are some things you can do to make your trip to the dietitian/diabetes educator as successful as possible.

- If you were asked to keep a food record or blood sugar log, bring those with you to the appointment. These logs help the educator establish patterns between your daily routine and how your blood sugar reacts to it. If you don't have a blood sugar log, bring your meter so it can be downloaded at the office. These records are important tools to managing your blood sugar and medication appropriately. Using your logs helps both you and the educator make diabetes fit into your lifestyle, rather than the other way around.

- Be honest. If you haven't been doing blood tests, or counting carbohydrates, or if you feel burned out, tell your educator. Honesty is the best way to establish a good relationship between you and your health care team. Together, you and your educator can create small, simple goals to help get you back on track. Even if your educator is not a person with diabetes, he or she can point you in the right direction to find the support you need.

- Ask questions and be engaged. As an educator, I can provide you with loads of great information and resources to help you on your way to excellent care. However, without your input, I don't know if these tools are useful for you. Asking questions and providing feedback also tells me you are interested. If you aren't interested, or don't find these resources helpful, tell me! I want to make sure I'm doing my best to help you. There's nothing wrong with taking charge of your education session and telling me exactly how I can help you better manage your diabetes.

Dieticians have very diverse training in the realm of dietetics, from learning about nutrients and how they work in the body, to the scientific properties of food. Especially for children, who are learning to manage diabetes on their own one day, this type of education can put them on a path to a lifetime of good food choices. Also, if you want to make a food item more blood sugar–friendly, consider giving your local dietitian a call! He or she can help you with recipe modifications and substitutions for your favorite dishes.

When it comes to best managing your diabetes, don't forget to include a registered dietitian. While not all dietitians have personal experience living with diabetes, we all strive to help you reach your goals. A dietitian is only successful when his or her patients are successful, too.

Courtney Slater is a Registered Dietitian and diabetes educator. She has a special interest in diabetes since she was diagnosed with type 1 diabetes at age 5. She shares her experiences on her blog, C's Life With D (www.cslifewithd.blogspot.com).

connected to food. The amount and type of foods eaten determine how much insulin is given at mealtimes. When blood sugar levels are low, we use food—often in the form of juice, candy, glucose tablets, or other quick-acting carbs—to bring that blood sugar back in range. When blood sugar is high, low- or no-carb snacks might be given to a hungry child instead of a regularly scheduled snack.

Food is also a central focus in many aspects of life. We celebrate birthdays with cake and ice cream. On Halloween, we go trick-or-treating, filling bags with candy. We put candy canes in Christmas stockings and hunt for plastic eggs filled with treats at Easter time. Almost every holiday we celebrate has a sweet food associated with it. There are two reasons why I think that children with diabetes should not be forbidden from partaking in such traditions.

First, these celebrations are part of being a kid in our society, and there's no better way to reinforce to your child that they are different than to tell them no. Second, given that diabetes care is so tied to food, the potential is great to create food issues that your child will struggle with for his or her entire life.

Of course, there are times when you will have to tell your child no to having certain high-carb foods. While I take the "everything in moderation" and "let them have cake" approach, I don't let my child eat anything she wants, any time she wants. It depends on the circumstances and/or the food. For instance, when we are at the bank and they offer her a lollipop, I might tell her to hold onto it

> ❗ When going to the movies, take an empty 4-cup plastic container. You can portion out your child's popcorn to make carb counting and portion control easier. Each 4-cup serving of popcorn has approximately 15 grams of carbs.

until later if it's not snack time. Quinn was even offered candy when she went with me to vote. Rather than getting upset about someone offering her candy and launching into an explanation that she has diabetes, I simply say thank you and tell her that we will save it for later. Because that's the routine, it's not upsetting for her. But if you have other children with you, you might tell them to do the same.

> **!** Your family probably eats the same foods over and over. Create a chart with serving sizes, carb counts, and carb factors for quick reference. Pin this list to a small corkboard mounted to the inside of an accessible cabinet or pantry door.

The preschool that Quinn attended, and our son now attends, has several great parties each year that take place between dinner and bedtime. One of the coveted activities is cookie or cupcake decorating. The fun is in the decorating, and that's not something I wanted to deny Quinn. At the first few parties after her diagnosis, she was still receiving injections. Having this treat would mean that she would need an extra injection. Because there were so many other activities for the kids to bounce around to, it was not a problem for Quinn to decorate her cookie or cupcake, and then move on to the next activity without eating. Instead, I wrapped up the treat and took it home so she could have it the next day with a meal, therefore avoiding the extra injection. When she began the insulin pump, this became a nonissue because giving an extra bolus is no big deal.

By restricting or forbidding some foods, you run the risk of making them even more tempting to your child. Make something completely off limits, and I guarantee that your child will seek it out. I have heard several stories from parents describing this exact phenomenon. One child was having blood sugar levels in the 300s, and the parents just couldn't figure out why. While doing laundry, they found wrappers in the child's pocket from candy that her friends had given her. Because candy was forbidden, she ate it secretly, without giving herself insulin. I personally feel that creating categories of off-limits foods can create dishonesty. A main theme of diabetes management that I see in adults is that you need to be honest with yourself in order to manage it effectively. It's our job as parents to foster good habits in our children so that they can make good choices as teens and, later, as adults.

> **!** If you like to store baking ingredients, cereals, and snacks in containers in your pantry, cut out the nutrition information label from the package and pop it into the container for quick reference.

What's worse: letting your child have candy or dessert once in a while with your knowledge or creating a scenario where your child feels the need to sneak certain foods? If you choose to allow your child to eat desserts and candy, they can be consumed at appropriate times with corresponding insulin. I have also found that including sweet treats as part of a meal lessens the blood sugar spike.

Sugar-Free Foods

Artificial sweeteners are something I never even considered giving my children before Quinn's diagnosis. In fact, I avoided them, choosing the least-refined sweeteners available. I bought snacks that were sweetened with evaporated cane juice rather than refined white sugar ... or worse, high-fructose corn syrup (HFCS). But when your child is diagnosed with type 1 diabetes, all bets are off. Well, not all of them. I reconsidered my stance against artificial sweeteners given that her choices were often something artificially sweetened or nothing. So how do you reconcile a firm belief that artificial ingredients are bad when there are times when sugar-free JELL-O or Kool-Aid is the only alternative? You give in a little.

That's something I've had to do a lot since her diagnosis. Now, I'm not saying that artificial sweeteners are free-flowing in our house—they are limited. The ironic thing is that my child never drank juice or Kool-Aid until after she was diagnosed. Now, she often has juice to treat lows and sometimes drinks half-strength sugar-free Kool-Aid or Crystal Light, but not all the time. She's even had sugar-free soda on rare occasions. I know another child with diabetes who is allowed to drink zero-carb soda all day long, and I can tell you all that caffeine is not good!

As part of our pump approval, we had to take a course in carb counting with a local dietician. We took the opportunity to talk with her about other things, including the use of artificial sweeteners. She stated that she would not be nervous giving our daughter artificial sweeteners *within reason.*

We've all heard tales that artificial sweeteners cause cancer in lab rats, right?

I used to tease a coworker who drank more than three liters of diet soda each day that he was producing formaldehyde and was slowly preserving himself from the inside!

> Sugar free does not mean carb free!

The Mayo Clinic website article "Artificial sweeteners: A safe alternative to sugar?" sheds some light on the acceptability of artificial sweeteners. *"People with diabetes may use artificial sweeteners because they make food taste sweet without raising blood*

OUR FAVORITE SNACK IDEAS

Free Snacks*
(5 Carbs Or Fewer)
1 popsicle made with sugar-free
   drink mix
1 sugar-free popsicle
3 celery sticks + 1 Tbs peanut
   butter
5 baby carrots
1 hard-boiled egg
1 cup cucumber slices + 1 Tbs
   ranch dressing
1/4 cup fresh blueberries
1 cup light popcorn
1/2 cup sugar-free JELL-O

Regular Snacks*
(10 to 20 Carbs Per Serving)
1 small apple
1 small orange
1/2 banana
1/2 cup unsweetened
   applesauce
4 oz. individual fruit cup
2 Tbs raisins
1 fruit roll-up
8 oz. or 1 carton light yogurt
4 oz. or 1/2 cup regular yogurt
1 yogurt tube (can freeze)

3/4 cup kefir
1/2 cup sugar-free pudding
1/2 cup lowfat ice cream
1 frozen fruit juice bar
1 1/2 graham crackers
4-5 vanilla wafers
5-6 saltine crackers
18 small pretzel twists
3 cups low-fat microwave popcorn
3 cups air poped popcorn
2 popcorn cakes
1/2 mini bagel with cream cheese
1/3 cup hummus + 1 cup
   raw veggies
1/4 cup cottage cheese + 1/2
cup canned or fresh fruit
1 cheese quesadilla (made with
   one 6-inch tortilla +
   1 oz. shredded cheese)
2 rice cakes + 1 Tbs peanut
   butter
5 whole wheat crackers + 1 piece
   of string cheese
1/2 turkey sandwich

*Read nutrition labels for exact
serving sizes and carb counts of
each food item.

sugar levels. But keep in mind that if you do have diabetes, some foods containing artificial sweeteners, such as sugar-free yogurt, can still affect your blood sugar level due to other carbohydrates or proteins in the food. Some foods labeled 'sugar-free'—such as sugar-free cookies and chocolates—may contain sweeteners, such as sorbitol or mannitol, which contain calories and can affect your blood sugar level. Some sugar-free products may also contain flour, which will raise blood sugar levels."

That's an important point to remember—sugar free does not mean carb free. I am sure that well-intentioned relatives and friends purchased sugar-free alternatives for your child after their diagnosis. Interestingly, certain brands of ice cream and whipped topping have *more* carbs in their sugar-free version than the regular recipes! That's all the more reason to read labels, not only for ingredients, but also for portion sizes and carb counts. Sugar-free foods can affect people with diabetes very differently. One family told me that their child's blood sugar spikes dramatically after having sugar-free syrup, while my daughter seems to do okay. Sometimes it's trial and error.

SUGAR ALCOHOLS—WATCH OUT ON LABELS

- sorbitol
- xylitol
- mannitol

While you are reading labels on sugar-free or reduced-sugar foods, take a look at the sugar alcohols, which are listed in the carbohydrates section, below the sugar. In some people, sugar alcohols can cause digestive issues, such as tummy aches and diarrhea. Children may be even more prone to these side effects. At a local diabetes walk, a d-dad had some sugar-free candy and warned Quinn not to eat too many. His daughter told us why … she ate too many and got the runs!

A Good Digital Scale—Worth Its Weight in Gold

In the beginning, when I was still overwhelmed, I ran out to the housewares store and bought a small, cheap scale to weigh out portions. You had to twist the little knob to get it to zero and then stare at tiny little lines to read how many ounces or grams the food weighed. The inaccuracy of this scale somewhat diminished the usefulness of the concept of weighing food to get a good carb count.

> Don't be afraid to ask. If I'm at the deli or at a restaurant, I always ask if they have nutritional information available. Deli items often come in a larger container that includes a food label.

Eventually I purchased a digital scale, which has improved my ability to accurately count carbs. The model we have is basic—you place a bowl or plate on top of the disc and it will measure in ounces or grams. You can even take it to zero between adding items to the dish. This no-frills scale serves its purpose well.

However, there is a Cadillac of digital scales that I've been looking at longingly on Internet shopping sites. These scales are pre-programmed with codes for different foods. You look up the code for a particular item and enter it into the keypad, and when you weigh the food, the screen looks like a nutrition label, listing the number of carbs for that portion. Magic!

These digital nutrition scales will cost you more—anywhere from $50 to $100—but may save you time and guesswork. Not only do they have a large database of foods, but many also allow you to program in custom foods, which is handy for recipes that you make often. A good digital scale will also come in handy when you use the carb-factor method, described on the next page.

Counting Carbs

In the hospital, we were given the option of using diabetic exchanges or counting carbs. Exchanges did not seem very accurate to me, whereas counting carbs is more systematic. It's the method that our family uses.

I've been teaching Quinn to read labels because it helps her make good choices about the foods she wants to eat. It's very common for her to pick up something at the grocery store, read the label, and shout "Mom, this has 16 carbs!" It always makes heads turn by people wanting to see what kind of child counts carbs. Even my non-diabetic son asks me how many carbs are in foods.

Reading the labels on packaged foods is relatively easy: look at the serving size or number of servings per package and the total carbohydrates per serving. That's why, in the beginning, we turned to packaged foods a lot. The portion sizes and carb counts were listed right there, so mealtime required less thinking. I remember that Quinn really liked eating a particular frozen meal for lunch that consisted of fish sticks, macaroni and cheese, and chocolate pudding. My mom, who served her lunch every weekday, called the number on the package to ask what the carb counts of the individual components were. The customer service

> **!** Counting the carbs in pasta presents its own challenge. The serving size in grams on nutritional labels is for the dry, uncooked pasta. The weight of cooked pasta can vary greatly based on how long it has cooked and how much water is absorbed. I weigh out the number of portions I am going to make using the dry weights. After cooking, I divide the total weight of the cooked pasta by the number of servings I made to get the weight of an individual serving.

rep was able to track down the information, and they even sent us some coupons!

After a while, we grew tired of a steady diet of packaged foods, and we missed some of our favorite recipes. It was time to get more adventurous.

Home-Cooked Meals and Recipes

I often get notes from readers of my D-Mom Blog saying they have relied on packaged foods, but would like to start cooking and baking again. It's a little intimidating at first; after all, there is enough to think about without having to do even *more* math at mealtime! But as time went on, I became more comfortable with figuring out the carbs in recipes and, yes, guessing carb counts when we were dining out or at someone's home.

> ! When measuring ingredients such as flour and sugar, which are high in carbs and can settle over time, weighing with a scale is more accurate for carb counting than using measuring cups.

When I make homemade anything, I count up the total carbs for the entire recipe, using all of the ingredients, and then divide that by the number of servings. For each of the individual ingredients, such as flour or sugar, I consult the labels and then weigh or measure, and then write down the carbs for that ingredient. For produce or other items that don't come with a nutritional label, I look them up in *The CalorieKing* book, website, or iPhone app.

So, you have added up all the individual components of the recipe and have a total carb count. How do you know how many carbs are in a serving? Some items are easy to divide into servings, while others are not. What I find helpful is to weigh the final product. Let's say that a recipe weighs a total of 568 grams, and the total carbs for the entire recipe is 122. If there are six servings, then each serving would weigh 95 grams and have 20 carbs. Another way to do the calculation is to use carb factors, described below.

> **!** Don't do the math twice. When you figure out the carbs for a recipe, either write out the portion size and carb counts right on the recipe or use a sticky note with the information.

Carb Factors

Using carb factors is the most precise way to count carbs. More and more I have been using carb factors because you aren't tied to a specific serving size. A carb factor is the percentage of a food by weight that is carbohydrate. The carb factor of a banana is 0.228. Let's figure out the number of carbs in a banana that weighs 100 grams: $100 \times 0.228 = 28.8$ carbs. If you looked up banana in a nutrition guide, you would have to estimate if it was a small, medium, or large banana and the number of carbs might be way off.

I often calculate carb factors using nutritional guides. *The Ultimate Guide to Carb Counting* by Gary Scheiner gives not only great explanations of how to count carbs, but also includes an extensive list of foods and their carb factors. Additionally, the USDA National Nutrient Database (www.nal.usda.gov/fnic/food-comp/search/) is a great resource. Look up the food you are going to eat, let's say Banana Nut Crunch cereal, which Randy and Quinn often have for breakfast. The database automatically sets a serving size as 100 grams (but also gives other serving size options). The carbohydrate value per 100 grams is 74.50. We slide the decimal to the left two places and the carb factor is 0.745. If Quinn

MAKE-AHEAD SMOOTHIES

Becka Siegel

If there's one healthy snack that never seems to go out of style with my kids, it's smoothies. Now, I'm not talking about the "wannabe" smoothies found at your local convenience store that are laden with sugary, artificial fruit-flavored syrup, but REAL smoothies, with REAL ingredients. Don't get fooled by the knockoffs!

Smoothies are one of the most versatile and foolproof things you can make. The possibilities are endless, and it's nearly impossible to mess them up. Smoothies are typically made of fruit, milk, protein powder, and ice; however, lots of other things can be added for extra flavor or nutrition

You can experiment to find a flavor your kids will love and ask for time and time again. Smoothies can also be frozen and eaten with a spoon. These are especially great for lunch boxes. Your kids' friends will be envious as they watch these frozen treats being devoured.

A few years ago, I invested in a Magic Bullet, which has paid for itself a hundred times over. In the warmer months, it has a permanent spot on my countertop since we tend to make smoothies on a daily basis during those times. They are oh-so-refreshing on a hot day! I like the Magic Bullet because it's much easier to clean up than a regular blender, and it's easier to make separate smoothies according to everyone's individual tastes. Of course, you don't need a Magic Bullet to make smoothies—an ordinary blender will do the trick, too.

I gather all my ingredients, get out four mugs and eight storage bowls, and can easily whip up eight one-cup smoothies in four different flavors in about five minutes. I pop the bowls in the freezer, and they're ready for a quick snack or to throw into a lunch box in the mornings. The smoothies will stay frozen until lunchtime and have a "hard ice cream" consistency. My kids are able to eat them with a heavy-duty plastic spoon and are always thrilled to see a smoothie in their lunch boxes!

Smoothies are also inexpensive. I buy fresh fruit or bags of frozen fruit, large tubs of plain or vanilla yogurt, and a can of protein powder, which lasts a very long time. I tend to make mostly yogurt-based smoothies; it's good for you and adds a nice creamy texture.

To keep track of the carbs for each smoothie serving, I add the total carbs of everything I'm putting into the blender and then divide the carbs according to how many servings I've made. I use a dry-erase marker to write the number of carbs on the lid of the bowl before placing them in the freezer.

Below, I have listed a few basic recipes to give you an idea of what goes into a typical smoothie, but you can vary it depending on your tastes. For extra health benefits, you can also add a teaspoon of wheat germ, brewer's yeast, and/or ground flaxseed. Also, if you prefer your smoothies a little sweeter, I recommend using regular or all-natural sugar, as opposed to an artificial sweetener or sugar alternative.

You also don't need to use yogurt in all of your smoothies. Instead, you can use milk, juice, or even water. These liquids help with the blending process. The only limit is your creativity. So, dust off those blenders and start whipping up some delicious smoothies today!

Strawberry-Banana
- 1 medium banana (I just break it in half)
- 1 cup fresh or frozen strawberries
- 1/2 cup plain or vanilla yogurt
- 1/2 cup milk
- 2 Tbs. protein powder (vanilla)
- 1 tsp. vanilla extract
- 3 ice cubes (optional)

Tropical Delight
- 1 medium banana
- 6 pineapple chunks
- 1 coconut popsicle
- 1/2 cup plain or vanilla yogurt
- 1/2 cup orange juice
- 2 Tbs. protein powder
- 3 ice cubes (optional)

continued on next page.

MAKE-AHEAD SMOOTHIES con't

Peachy Keen

- 1 cup fresh or frozen peaches
- 1 cup plain or vanilla yogurt
- 1/2 cup milk
- 1/4 tsp. nutmeg
- 2 Tbs. protein powder
- 1/2 tsp. almond extract (optional)
- 3 ice cubes (optional)

Becka Siegel is the parent of Brandon, who was diagnosed with type 1 diabetes in June of 2002 at the age of 6. She writes the blog Just a Bunch of Momsense (www.justabunchofmomsense.com), where she shares a variety of things including recipes, gift ideas, DIY projects, useful tips on diabetes, couponing and more, but mostly focuses on healthy, diabetes-friendly lunchbox ideas, suitable for kids, teens, and adults.

pours a bowl of cereal that weighs 45 grams, we multiply that by 0.745 and see that it has 33.5 carbs.

You may ask why I didn't just enter in a 1-gram portion. I have found that it can create huge variances when you do the math on larger portion sizes, particularly of higher-carb foods. Depending on your child's insulin-to-carb ratio, this can make a noticeable difference in the size of the bolus!

To figure out the carb factor for packaged foods, divide the total carbs for a single serving by the weight in grams of that one serving. If a serving of fish crackers has 20 carbs and weighs 30 grams, the carb factor is 20/30 or 0.666.

It's not difficult to figure out the carb factor on recipes, either.

And remember, when you do the math the first time, write it down so you don't have to do it again. Add up the carbs from ALL of the ingredients used in the recipe and divide this by the total weight of the cooked product. When I added up the ingredients in the chili recipe I cook often, it had 122 carbs. I weighed the cooked chili in a large bowl using my digital scale, and it weighed 568 grams. So 122 carbs divided by 568 gives us a carb factor of 0.215. Using this calculation, you will see that if you have a serving that weighs 95 grams and you multiply that by the carb factor of 0.215, it has 20 carbs. Using the carb factor, you don't have to always serve the same portion. If Quinn wants a bowl of chili that weighs, say, 75 grams, then it will have 75 x 0.215 or 16 carbs.

In the appendix at the end of the book, I've included a list of carb factors for some common foods.

Dining Out

As our very first restaurant experience after diagnosis illustrates, you can't always count on a restaurant to have nutrition information available. I can't tell you the number of times I have asked for it and have been told they have it on their website, yet they aren't willing to look it up for me. However, I am finding that more and more restaurants have the information available in either a brochure you can take with you, on a chart posted on the wall, or in a binder in the office that you can look at.

I have several tools for counting carbs while dining at restaurants or getting take-out food. First, if I know ahead of time that we are going to a particular restaurant, I will look at their website. I can either write down the carb counts of several menu items that I think Quinn might choose or download the PDF of their guide.

Second, when I'm at restaurants I ask if they have a nutrition guide that I can have. If it's a restaurant we go to frequently, I take it home with me for future reference. Third, if it's a restaurant that doesn't have information available in-house and I didn't look it up ahead of time, I will access their website using my smartphone.

I developed a chart using a spreadsheet that lists the restaurants we frequent and the food items that Quinn usually eats. The printed copy hangs on the bulletin board that's mounted on the back of our pantry door for quick reference when we have takeout. I also keep a PDF of this file on my phone. Using apps like iDisk and Dropbox, I have saved not only my restaurant cheat sheet, but also guides that I have downloaded from restaurants. I can also pull up The CalorieKing app on my phone. This app lists many specific restaurants and also enables you to search generically for a food item. As a last resort, you can take a good guess as to the number of carbs in a meal. You will find that the longer you count carbs, the better you'll get at estimating.

An added issue is that restaurants may not give you the exact portion size for which the nutritional information was calculated. Do you really think that bag of fries is the right weight? I personally find it excessive to bring a food scale into restaurants to weigh out portions, but some families do find this to be a useful tool.

Currently, the FDA is considering nutrition-disclosure standards or menu labeling regulations for restaurants that may be in place by mid-2012. According to the FDA's website, *"The law will require restaurants with 20 or more locations to provide calories on menus and menu boards, and make other written nutrition information available upon request."* I have noticed that some large chains are already posting calories on their menu boards; if only they would also post carbs!

Snacks

Depending on your child's age and type of insulin therapy, your medical care team may suggest a number of daily snacks, either with or without insulin to cover the carbs. It's common for younger children who are on injections to have several uncovered snacks each day, including mid-morning and mid-afternoon, as the insulin bolus from the previous meal peaks. In addition, a bedtime snack that includes protein to keep blood sugar levels even overnight is often recommended. As children get older, many begin eliminating snacks or covering them with insulin, particularly if they are on an insulin pump since it would not require an extra injection.

Generally, suggested snacks are a serving size of about 15 grams of carbs. If a child is hungry between mealtimes, or if blood sugar levels are higher than a certain threshold as determined by the medical team, a child might eat a "free" snack, which has 5 grams of carbs or less. The thinking is that

> **!** When opening a box of snacks, take a few minutes to portion them out. That way, you don't have to weigh or count out a serving next time.

5 grams of carbs will not affect blood sugar levels drastically. Since protein slows the peak of carbohydrates, bedtime snacks include 5 or more grams of protein.

While many snacks served to kids are sugary or high in carbs, I think you will find that there is a long list of snacks your child can enjoy. Quinn does have her share of vanilla wafers, pretzel twists, and cheddar bunnies, but she also enjoys fresh and dried fruit, homemade smoothies, cheese and crackers, hummus and pita chips or celery sticks, frozen yogurt tubes, and a large variety of other snacks. The possibilities are endless. Remember that some

IT'S ALL IN THE TIMING

Gary Scheiner MS, CDE

In most cases, mealtime (bolus) insulin doses are based on three things: the amount of carbohydrates, the pre-meal blood sugar, and whether or not exercise will take place. But there is a fourth dimension, *time*, that must be taken into account. The timing of a bolus can make or break its effectiveness: just like a baseball player who must swing the bat so that it crosses the plate at the same exact moment as the ball. Swing too early or too late and you're going to strike out. Bolus too early or too late and your blood sugar is going to do a lot of bouncing around.

Enter Glycemic Index

Glycemic Index (GI) refers to the rate at which carbohydrates convert into blood glucose. While virtually all carbohydrates convert into blood glucose eventually, some convert much faster than others. Pure glucose is given a GI score of 100; everything else is compared to the digestion/absorption rate of glucose. For example, baked potatoes have a GI of 85, wheat bread is 68, spaghetti is 41, and yogurt is only 33.

What the numbers represent is the percentage of carbohydrate that turns into blood glucose in the first two hours after eating that food. Foods with a high GI (greater than 70) tend to digest and convert to blood glucose the fastest, with a significant blood glucose "peak" occurring in 30 to 45 minutes. Foods with a moderate GI (45–70) digest a bit slower, resulting in a less-pronounced blood glucose peak approximately one to one and a half hours after they are consumed. Foods with a low GI (below 45) tend to make a gradual appearance in the bloodstream. The blood glucose peak is usually quite modest and may take several hours to occur.

Most starchy foods (rice, potato, cereal, bread) have a relatively high GI; they are digested easily and convert into blood glucose quickly. Exceptions include starches found in pasta and legumes, which break down slowly. Foods with dextrose in them, such as glucose tablets, tend to have a very high GI and are thus well suited for treating hypoglycemia. Fructose (fruit sugar) and lactose (milk sugar) are a bit slower to convert into blood glucose. Table sugar (sucrose) has a moderate GI. Foods that contain fiber or large amounts of fat tend to have lower GIs than foods that do not.

What Is It Good For?

Why is glycemic index important? Because the effect of dietary carbohydrates is what really matters. Knowing the glycemic index of a food helps in determining the optimal time to take the mealtime insulin. For foods with a high GI (greater than 70), it is best to take mealtime rapid-acting insulin 20 to 30 minutes prior to eating. This will allow the insulin peak to coincide as closely as possible with the blood sugar peak. Taking insulin for high-GI foods just before or while eating would produce a significant after-meal blood sugar spike, as the insulin would lag behind the blood sugar rise by about half an hour or more.

For foods with a moderate GI (approximately 45–70), as well as most "mixed" meals, it is usually best to take mealtime insulin five to ten minutes prior to eating. With low-GI (below 45) foods, taking insulin prior to eating is likely to lead to hypoglycemia about one hour later, followed by a delayed blood sugar rise. Instead, take the insulin right *after* eating. A second option is to split the rapid-acting insulin into two parts: half given with the meal, the other half about an hour later. A third option, available to insulin pump users, is to program the dose at the beginning of the meal but extend the delivery over 60 to 90 minutes.

How Precise Is the Timing?

Of course, nothing having to do with diabetes is simple. The after-meal blood sugar rise is affected by more than just the glycemic index. Physical activity and stress tend to slow down digestion. Low blood sugar, on the other hand, accelerates the rate of digestion. Even glycemic index can vary from person to person, and there's really no way of knowing how different food mixtures will react. What glycemic index is good for is *categorizing* foods according to their relative impact: fast, moderate, and slow.

continued on next page.

IT'S ALL IN THE TIMING con't

When looking at complete meals, the main source of carbohydrate should dictate the rate of blood glucose rise. For example, a meal where pasta is the primary carbohydrate should be treated as low-GI. A meal where potato is the major source of carbs should be treated as high-GI. Timing the boluses accordingly will give you an advantage when it comes to stabilizing the after-meal blood sugar. And given the variables we have to contend with on a daily basis, we can use every advantage we get!

Gary Scheiner MS, CDE is Owner and Clinical Director of Integrated Diabetes Services (www.integrateddiabetes.com) and Dean of Type 1 University (www.type1university.com). He is the author of several books, including Think Like A Pancreas: A Practical Guide to Managing Diabetes with Insulin. Gary has had type 1 diabetes since 1985. He and his staff offer diabetes management consulting services throughout the world via phone and the internet.

higher-carb foods might not be good choices, mainly because a 15-carb serving might not be filling.

Individual Snack Packs

Many of the 100-calorie packs that you see in the grocery store now have approximately 15 grams of carbs. That seems like a great choice, and I've been known to buy them when I'm in a hurry. However, these 100-calorie packs are very expensive per serving, and you are paying for the packaging. Instead, I make my own 15-carb snack packs.

Once every week or two, I take a few minutes to make up a large batch of snack packs. I gather boxes of snacks, small containers and snack-size plastic bags, a bowl to measure in, and my scale. So that I don't have to do math every time, I have a note posted on the back of the cabinet door where we keep our snacks that has the weight of a 15-gram serving of the snacks we frequently purchase. I weigh out the portions, putting them into containers or plastic bags, and toss them into our snack box.

At the beginning of the school week, I grab ten of the snack packs and put them in Quinn's lunch box that is designated for her snacks. Appropriately, the lunch box features Scooby-Doo enjoying a Scooby Snack! My kids, even the one without diabetes, can go to the snack box and make a selection on their own at snack time. Your child with diabetes might be having 14 regular snacks, plus seven bedtime snacks every week, so this preportioned method can really reduce your work.

My kids are yogurt junkies, and I don't like purchasing the small cups of yogurt geared toward kids because they have added sugar, are unnatural in color, and are just plain expensive. Not to mention that those little cups adorned with the characters kids love are just extra packaging. I usually buy yogurt in a big tub and divvy it up. I find that if I divide it into my own storage containers right when it's opened, it saves me time and energy in the future. In other words, my individual yogurt cups are just as easy as those convenient kids' cups.

> ! Use a dry-erase marker to write the number of carbs when dividing foods such as yogurt and applesauce into small plastic containers. The marker can easily be wiped away before washing.

Buying by the large tub is better for the environment because there is less packaging, and it is better for your wallet because it's

Keep a stash with you. I keep a container of nonperishable 15-carb snacks in the car.

much cheaper per ounce.

To tell you the truth, my kids can't get enough of it. You can also buy larger containers of natural applesauce for this reason.

The easiest way to portion yogurt and applesauce is to get out that handy digital scale. Using measuring cups is messy and only requires more cleanup. You can purchase small, colorful containers in the toddler section at the store, and then weigh out portions of yogurt or applesauce into the individual cups using a spoon. I do this assembly line–style. I usually portion out the weight equivalent to a half-cup serving.

THE CELIAC CONNECTION

Jennie Rallison

Shortly after my daughter Brittany was diagnosed with type 1 diabetes I noticed her common complaint of tummy aches. She spent a lot of time in the bathroom, and after eating meals she would be doubled over with stomach pain. I attributed it to the diabetes and asked her endocrinologist why it made her stomach hurt. He simply replied that we should check her for celiac disease, as it is quite common for kids with type 1 to have it as well. At the time, we were extremely overwhelmed with her diabetes diagnosis and daily care, so I didn't even bother to ask what celiac was. I was on a need-to-know basis, so I figured we'd let them do the blood draw and worry about it only if we had to. A week went by when it dawned on me to follow up with the doctor and see what the results were. Sure enough, the blood work indicated she had celiac disease, and a stomach biopsy confirmed the finding.

Celiac disease is an autoimmune disorder, just like type 1 diabetes.

THE CELIAC CONNECTION con't

In fact, according to the American Diabetes Association, about one in twenty people with diabetes also have celiac disease. With celiac, the body is not able to process gluten, which is found in the protein in barley, wheat and rye. Brittany's body was literally attacking itself inside her intestines, killing the villi or fingerlike projections that absorb food and nutrients. There is nothing that could have prevented her body from having it, and unfortunately, just as with diabetes, there is no cure. The only way to treat celiac disease is to eat gluten free, and over time, the body will heal itself.

So, we set out on another life-altering journey to modify Brittany's diet to now be gluten free. I was already struggling with measuring, carb counting and dosing every little bite of food she ate. Now, I would be forced to carefully read every food label for ingredients that contained gluten. The diabetes didn't necessarily change her diet. We were already conscious to balance protein and carbs to sustain better blood sugar, but eating gluten free severely limited her food choices. Gone were the days of quick and convenient stops at a drive-through window and store-bought convenience foods like granola bars.

We quickly learned that sticking to a simple diet of meats, veggies, and fruits without anything added was a safe way to eat. Luckily, Brittany enjoyed a healthy diet, so she didn't feel like she was being quite so limited. In the first couple years of her diagnosis, we had to buy many of her gluten-free foods at a specialty store, and they cost about three times as much for a third of the quantity. However, in the past few years more name-brand food manufacturers have embraced the need for gluten-free options, allowing us to find many products at our corner grocery store. Many restaurants are also offering gluten-free menu options, as well as training their staff on cross contamination. There seem to be new options every day, and I am excited for her to have choices and variety in her diet.

In our home, we do not solely eat gluten free, though most of our meals are gluten free. I tend to buy cereals that are gluten free and often make treats without gluten. For us, it comes down to a cost factor, as we

continued on next page.

THE CELIAC CONNECTION con't

are a family of six living on a budget. Food prep and storage also require special considerations. I boil her rice noodles separately from our spaghetti, and only she gets to eat the expensive gluten-free bread. Brittany has her own shelf in the pantry with her own toaster, strainer, and bakeware. I stock our favorite gluten-free food items, snacks, and specialty flours there, as well as certified gluten-free oats. This shelf is up above the other shelves so crumbs don't fall on her items. I am careful to have clean working areas in the kitchen and prepare her meals first. At family get-togethers, we allow her to dish up her food first to avoid someone inadvertently putting a spoon from a gluten-filled dish into an item that was gluten free.

It is definitely a daily task to ensure that her meals are gluten free. Food is a factor almost everywhere you go. Although it can be a hassle to go out to eat or to a party, at least there is a treatment, and she is able to enjoy these things. I will never forget walking out of the hospital after Brittany's initial stay for the diabetes diagnosis and being grateful that she was still a walking, talking, fully functional child. While diabetes and celiac disease are life-changing, she is still able to participate in all that life has to offer her.

Jennie Rallison is the parent of Brittany, who was diagnosed with type 1 diabetes at the age of 7 and also celiac disease at the age of 8. She is the blog author of Gluten Free Eating (www.eatglutenfreelikeme.blogspot.com) where she shares her family's gluten-free recipes and tips.

CHAPTER SEVEN

Less Stress, More Happiness

With all the added tasks and concerns we have as parents of a child with diabetes, it's easy to get caught up in the details of daily management and lose sight of the fact that your child is still a child—with all the enthusiasm and curiosity that entails. He or she may have diabetes, but it's important for long-term well being to have normal childhood experiences. Playtime, parties, holidays, and sports are supposed to be fun but, let's face it, diabetes adds a challenge to these rites of childhood. So, how do you balance caring for your child's health and letting them just be kids? I have a few suggestions.

Putting Diabetes in the Background

Your child has diabetes, but is diabetes all your child is? Of course not. It's our job as parents to make sure our d-kids can be the kids they are meant to be, without making diabetes a burden they must think about every minute of the day. Diabetes needs to become background noise. Yes, your child needs to have their blood sugar checked and get insulin, but these should become minor interruptions, not the most prominent events each day.

Your attitude toward diabetes will likely be the attitude your child adopts. If you're relaxed, your child will be relaxed. If you're high strung, you better believe your child will become stressed about diabetes, too!

I personally don't like my daughter to start her day thinking about her diabetes. I know you have those 15 seconds every morning, before you hear your child stir, when you wonder if she's still alive in there. I get it. It's scary. But does she need to start her day like that?

When your child comes into your room or meets you downstairs in the kitchen, don't let the first questions out of your mouth be "Did you check your blood sugar? What was your number?" You'll get to that in a few minutes. If they are walking and talking and not telling you that they feel low, then it can wait. Instead, ask them how they slept, let them tell you about their dreams, or ask them what they're excited about for the day. In other words, start the day on a positive note.

The same goes for after school. If your child had blood sugar issues during the school day, I'm sure the nurse or other staff already called you. When your child comes out into the schoolyard, you can see they're just fine. Unless they feel low, resist the urge to immediately check their blood sugar. Let them linger with their friends for a few minutes or play on the playground. Don't let the first questions you ask be "What was your lunchtime number? Did you remember to test when you were supposed to? Did you eat all of your lunch?" Instead, ask how your child's day was.

Every day, during the drive home, my daughter tells me three things about her school day. It makes her feel like I care about her day and keeps me informed about what's going on at school. If any of her three things have to do with diabetes, and they usually don't, it's because she wanted to tell me about it, not because I put an emphasis on it. Quinn may test her blood sugar in the car as we drive or when we arrive back home, but it's not the focus of our chitchatting.

When you arrive home and your child throws down his or her backpack while running through the house to the backyard, that's the time to get out the meter or logbook and look at the numbers from the day. You can follow up in a little while if you have questions about their blood sugar levels or how much insulin the child received.

Playdates and Sleepovers

How many times have you heard, "Mom, can we have a playdate?" I'll admit that it really saddened me to watch children pair up after school and go home with friends, because I couldn't just send my daughter home with just anyone. When Quinn started asking for playdates, I always suggested that the other child come to our house. I found it easier to have the playdate at our house because I didn't have to think about training or worry about her. However, as with all things in life, your child needs to have some experiences without you.

When you get to know the other families at school, you might develop a relationship with a parent whom you would trust with your child's care. Perhaps a parent has a medical background, is a teacher, or child-care provider. Maybe they are just willing to learn the basics of diabetes care.

Keep your ears open, because you might just find other families with firsthand knowledge of diabetes. Are there other children with diabetes at school who might be friends with your child? We know children at school who have siblings, parents, or close relatives with type 1 diabetes.

When training other families, you don't have to instruct them as fully as you would the school nurse or other staff. You just need to teach them enough so that they can care for your child, including giving an appropriate snack, checking blood sugar, and when they might need to use glucagon and call 911. Depending on the age of your child, she will likely be able to do many of the tasks herself. Sometimes I send a snack so I know she gets the right amount of carbs.

I find it useful to print out my instruction sheet that includes the symptoms of low and high blood sugar and how to treat them and what to do in case of a severe low. Remember that you are just a phone call away. I make myself available by phone whenever Quinn is in someone else's care. If you are really reluctant to let your child be in someone else's care, but want to give them the experience of being away from home, plan playdates at locations such as the library, a park, or the mall so your child can be supervised by the other parent but you are still close by.

! Adopt a "buddy system" for playing in the neighborhood.
● Teach a friend what to look for if your child's blood sugar drops, and instruct them to run to your home or call you for help.

The only sleepovers Quinn has had, so far, have been at her grandparents' house. While these, in theory, are diabetes-free nights for me, my mother does call to confirm boluses for meals and snacks and if/when to check blood sugar overnight. Sometimes Quinn's blood sugar inexplicably goes high when staying the night. We have looked at all possible causes, from pet allergies to an adrenaline rush from the excitement. However, on one occasion that was heartbreaking for Quinn, I just had to bring her home to deal with a really high, very stubborn blood sugar. But she keeps having these sleepovers because it's good to have time away from her brother and parents and spend time alone with her grandparents.

Sleepovers present similar challenges to playdates. You need to find families you trust, who are willing to be trained in your child's care. The older and more self dependent your child is, the easier sleepovers will be. Children who are already checking their own blood sugar, counting carbs, and figuring out boluses at school can do these tasks at sleepovers, calling parents to confirm the decisions and calculations they have made. If your child routinely gets a blood sugar check during the night, you can enlist the parents to set their alarm and call you if it is above or below a certain range of numbers.

For younger children who need more assistance, there are several options if the friend's parents aren't well versed in diabetes

PLAYDATE TIPS

- Teach, but don't over-train other parents. While you want them to be knowledgeable, you don't want to scare them off.
- Include an instruction sheet that highlights symptoms of low and high blood sugar and how to treat them.
- Show the parents the contents of the d-supply bag so that they know what the blood sugar meter looks like and where you keep the juice and glucagon.
- Send an appropriate snack or give a list of common snacks and portion sizes.
- Remind them that you are only a phone call away and won't mind being called even for what might seem like something trivial.
- Breathe.

care. You can pop over at dinnertime and bedtime to count carbs, check blood sugar, and give insulin. The parents can do the overnight checks and call or text you. Alternatively, a child can participate in all aspects of the sleepover, including getting into pajamas and reading a bedtime story, and you can pick the child up to sleep at home, maybe even returning them in time for breakfast. If your child is ready for sleepovers, but you aren't quite ready to let them spend the night at someone else's house, you can always invite friends to your home for a pajama party.

Birthday Parties

There are several issues with birthday parties—the food, the activity, and the supervision. I've told you my philosophy that children need to be children, and that includes going to birthday parties, as well as eating cake and ice cream. Some parents may ask you ahead of time if they should make any accommodations for your child. I personally don't use a lot of artificial sweeteners and try to stay away from sugar alcohols. I would rather Quinn eat the same foods as the other children at the party and then give the appropriate insulin for it. Not to mention that sugar-free ice cream usually has more carbs than regular! I always let Quinn have the cake and ice cream, and maybe some of the other goodies that are served, and then give a bolus for the estimated number of carbs that she eats. Where I usually draw the line is with the beverages. I typically ask her to have water, or I will send along a low-carb drink pouch, instead of letting her drink punch or other sugary drinks, which I know will spike her blood sugar. Eat the cake, skip the drink. Birthday cake is totally bolus-worthy, and I know Quinn never minded getting that extra injection when she was on multiple daily injections.

Many of the parties we host and go to have some type of physical activity involved. We held her most recent birthday party at the facility where she takes gymnastics. When it was time to eat cupcakes, she actually needed to get some carbs in her since the kids had been so active. Adrenaline from all the excitement can also raise blood sugar. Depending on the type of activity, your child might need a blood sugar check or two.

COUNTING CARBS AT PARTIES

Pizza (average slice) - 30 carbs

Cupcake with icing - 30 carbs

Medium piece of cake with icing (not too big, not too small, and definitely not a corner piece) - 30 carbs

½ **cup of vanilla ice cream (a decent size scoop)** - 15 carbs

Punch too many carbs!

Your biggest obstacle at parties probably has nothing to do with carb counting and everything to do with freedom. Just as with playdates, you have to decide if you are comfortable leaving your child in someone else's care. A playdate where the parent has to oversee only a small number of children is different than a party with 15 eight-year-olds running around. If the parent is one who has already taken care of your child, then you might feel comfortable dropping your child off and leaving. Remember, you are only a phone call away. But you may feel better staying. In fact, many parents appreciate the extra set of hands. You can either be right there participating in the party or you can bring a book to read and sit on the sidelines, only interacting when needed to give insulin and check blood sugar. I have done it both ways.

The key to birthday parties is to let them have fun and keep diabetes from taking center stage. Yes, test blood sugar and give insulin as needed, but let your kid play with his or her friends and partake in the festivities. And if you underestimated the number of carbs in that cake, it's not the end of the world. I check Quinn's blood sugar about two hours after she has cake and give her a correction with insulin if needed.

Happier Holidays

In the first few months after my daughter's diagnosis, I remember lamenting that she and her grandmother wouldn't be able to carry on their tradition of baking cookies. What a foolish thought. Of course she can bake cookies! Food is entrenched in nearly every holiday, and I know that it can be daunting, but I remind myself that all things, including holiday sweets and treats, can be consumed in moderation.

Admittedly, we restricted our children's consumption of candy before the diagnosis, so my daughter's expectations about how many sweets she could have at Easter or Halloween didn't send her into protest. But a surefire way to make your child feel different because of their diabetes is to treat him or her differently than your other children or classmates.

Easter: The Thrill of the Hunt

On Easter, our focus is on fun. The Easter Bunny leaves a note for the kids with clues as to where he hid surprises. The kids grab their Easter baskets and follow the clues. At each location there is one item for each child. These include non-food items such as a book, sidewalk chalk, a toy car, or small plastic animal, plastic eggs filled with coins, and, of course, it culminates in finding a chocolate bunny!

I know your first thought was of that chocolate bunny. Kids delight in getting a chocolate bunny. The key is not letting them eat it all at once. When we let Quinn have a little chocolate as dessert over the next week, we break off a piece of it and weigh it, using carb factors to calculate how many carbs in each piece. (Refer to the section on carb factors.)

> ! Set limits up front. "I'll let you have a plate of holiday food, but let's save the cupcake for later." "You can have two pieces of candy tonight, but let's pick out your ten favorite pieces to have over the coming weeks."

We also go to a big Easter egg hunt in our town every year. I treat it similarly to Halloween, allowing her a few treats over the next few days, and then getting rid of the rest of the stash. While a big part of Easter celebrations is the candy, you will find that it's more about the thrill of the hunt.

Halloween: The Trick to Treats

Halloween is one of our family's favorite holidays. We begin scoping out the decorations the minute they appear on store shelves. We visit multiple pumpkin patches to buy pumpkins and gourds, and attend several parties. We go trick-or-treating in our neighborhood, and even at a nearby zoo. Sometimes we even have more than one costume per person because the kids invent them from clothes in their closets and our dress-up stash.

So what's our trick to dealing with treats? Don't make the treats the focus.

At one of our yearly parties, the tradition is for kids to decorate large cupcakes with mounds of frosting and sugar sprinkles. When our daughter was on multiple daily injections, we didn't want her eating this right before her bedtime blood sugar check, and we didn't want yet another injection. So, we let her partake in the decorating to her heart's content, and then we popped the creation in a container we had brought with us for her to consume the next day at mealtime. Now that she's on an insulin pump, she eats without worrying about that extra injection. The point is that the fun is often in the process. Decorating the cupcake is the fun activity, and once she was finished with it, she ran off to the next station.

> ! Go through your child's stash of Halloween candy and pull out items that are good for treating low blood sugar such as Smarties, Skittles, Swedish Fish, and other low-fat, high-sugar items.

Long before the diagnosis, we began handing out small containers of Play-Doh and various trinkets such as pencils, spider rings, bouncy balls, and plastic skeletons to trick-or-treaters. Kids love these goodies. Setting an example that treats don't have to be candy might catch on with the neighbors. And the best part is, if there are leftovers, you can stash them away for next year.

But don't tell your child with diabetes that they can't eat the mound of candy that was collected on All Hallow's Eve. Instead, decide on the number of pieces that can be eaten each day as dessert after a meal so there isn't an extra injection. Of course they can indulge in a piece or two on Halloween night. It's also a good idea to have the same rules for all your family members. If everyone is limited, then your child won't feel like they are being singled out.

One Halloween, my daughter went low while we were out

haunting the neighborhood. She asked if she could have a piece of candy, and I figured why not. Later, I read the labels and realized that both Smarties and glucose tabs have the same first ingredient: dextrose. Now I keep a supply of Smarties in our pantry because

> **!** Consider donating leftover candy to food pantries, the pediatric ward at the hospital, or organizations that send candy to soldiers serving overseas.

they are cheaper and a lot more fun! I go through the kids' candy stash and pull out items that are good for treating lows, such as Smarties and Skittles. Some doctors do not recommend chocolate for treating hypoglycemia because the fat content makes it slower to absorb.

I just had to laugh at my non-diabetic child one Halloween. When Rowan was three years old, he yelled, "Yes! Smarties!" every time he received one. It's not the most indulgent candy in the world (I personally prefer peanut butter cups), but it was the only candy he knew by name!

December Holidays

No matter what holiday you celebrate in December, there is bound to be indulgent food at every family get-together and party. As with the other holidays, an "all things in moderation" approach will let your child celebrate while not feeling differentiated.

I was actually surprised to find that some of the traditional Christmas treats, such as Advent calendar chocolates, candy canes, and even Pez aren't that high in carbs. The Advent calendars I picked up the last few years from the drugstore have tiny little chocolates with only two carbs each—all the fun, none of the

> For pure sugar candy such as candy canes, 1 gram weight equals 1 gram of carbs. If your child wants a candy cane and you don't have the package, weigh it for a good estimate. Granulated table sugar also has 1 gram carb per gram weight.

bolus! Anything under five carbs is considered a free food and can be given without corresponding insulin. Of course, if Quinn eats her daily nibble of Christmas chocolate as her dinner dessert, I'll tack on the two carbs. But this is one holiday indulgence she can enjoy without giving a second thought to managing her diabetes.

Alternatively, I found a sticker Advent countdown at a local specialty toy store. I have also seen Lego and Playmobil countdown calendars, though they are a bit pricey. My kids love the anticipation of Christmas, and what's a better way to help them count down than with an Advent calendar, even if it has chocolates, stickers, or some other treat?

One year, the kids kept asking for candy canes because they had never tried them. Some companies do make sugar-free or artificially sweetened candy canes, but you know my take on it: I try to avoid sugar alcohols and prefer the real thing with insulin to cover it. So, I purchased some mini candy canes. Three candy canes had 13 grams of carbs, which is approximately 4 grams of carbs each. Not bad! And you know what happened? Each kid had a couple of candy canes and then forgot about them. I found them at the back of the cabinet almost a year later and tossed them out.

Another year, a family member wanted to give our kids Pez. I said no because it was just more sugar to keep Quinn from over consuming. But I bet everyone reading this got Pez in his or her stocking as a child. Oh, the characters! Oh, the little tablets of pure sugar that tasted like absolutely nothing, but for some reason were so fun to eat. So, as I was shopping for stocking stuffers, I came across the display of Pez and actually turned over the package and read the label. Each roll, which has 12 pieces, has only 9 grams of carbs. That's 0.75 grams of carbs in each piece, which is not bad at all. Again, everything in moderation.

JUST AS SWEET

Here are some alternatives to candy for holidays and parties:

Easter

Hot Wheels or Matchbox cars

My Little Pony or Littlest Petshop

Books

Puzzles

Sidewalk chalk

Bubbles

Plastic eggs filled with a handful
 of change

Halloween

Eyeball bouncy balls

Rubber bracelets

Skull and spider rings

Pencils

Erasers in fun shapes

Rubber bats

Temporary tattoos

Stickers

Play-Doh

Christmas Stocking Stuffers

Lip balm

Cars or plastic pets (like Easter)

Mittens or gloves

Stickers

Activity packs

Card games

Holiday pencils and erasers

Fresh fruit such as apples or oranges

Sports and Exercise Strategies

Quinn is very active in sports, and I have come to understand that not all sports are created equally when it comes to diabetes management. The strategies that work for one sport might have

> ! • Take advantage of regularly scheduled breaks during recreational activities. Use the time when the Zamboni cleans the ice or during hourly pool checks to do a quick blood sugar check and give a snack, if needed.

the opposite effect for another. Although it's intuitive that you need less insulin during exercise because the body uses glucose for fuel, this hasn't always been the case for us.

When Quinn goes to dance and gymnastics, we follow the oft-given advice to have a snack of 15 carbs before beginning the exercise. These classes are one hour long. Sometimes this is enough to get her through the class, and sometimes she still goes low. I have also found that even if Quinn's blood sugar is in range after her late afternoon gymnastics class, and she's in range at dinner and again at bedtime, sometimes she's low in the middle of the night. I now know that on gymnastics nights, I need to do a couple of overnight blood sugar checks.

Thirty minutes of roller skating plummets her blood sugar, and I know I have to give her a snack before and test afterward, usually following up with another snack. But sometimes she can ice-skate nonstop for a three-hour public skate, and her blood sugar stays even. While she's ice-skating, I normally check her at each of the Zamboni breaks and treat accordingly.

Some days during soccer camp in 100-degree heat, Quinn was sucking down Gatorade and popping grapes in her mouth as if she had a working pancreas, barely keeping her blood sugar at the low end of her range. Yet other days, she didn't go low. Since there was no way to know how her body would react to a three-hour-a-day soccer camp in July heat, I checked her blood sugar often and reacted as needed.

And then we have the six weeks of daily swim lessons that my kids take in the early evening each summer. As I had always been instructed to do, I would give Quinn 15 grams of carbs before swimming, only to be shocked and horrified that as she toweled off a number in the 300s would pop up on her meter! For some kids, swimming makes blood sugar tank—but not for my child. The endocrinologist suggested that instead of giving Quinn 15 grams of uncovered carbs before swimming, we give her 20 carbs and bolus for half. The doctor explained that swimming uses large muscle groups and that her body may not have been effectively using her glucose stores during the activity. Giving her a little larger snack with a small amount of insulin would enable the body to use the glucose. This strategy seems to work well for us.

The key to dealing with sports is to figure out how your child's body reacts to each sport they play and develop a proactive game plan. But you need to be flexible, because the body may not react to exercise the same way each time. Other factors, such as insulin that is still working from the most recent bolus, rebound from low blood sugar earlier in the day, and even weather can affect your little athlete's body.

> ! Take your own sugar-free hot cocoa mix to the ice rink.
>
> ● The snack bar is usually happy to give you a cup of hot water to mix your own, especially if you are purchasing other items.

Your Diabetes Science Experiment written by Ginger Vieira, who has type 1 diabetes and is a champion power lifter, is a good resource to look to if sports have you scratching your head. Ginger describes "experiments" that will help you understand certain causes of low and high blood sugar and how to avoid them. Ginger says: "*By realizing that there is a reason behind every single number I see on my meter, any high or low blood sugar no longer leads me to feeling angry, frustrated, or discouraged. When I can explain those numbers clearly using true facts of how my body functions, and then actually adjust my insulin and nutrition to prevent those unwanted numbers from happening again, I have much greater control over how diabetes impacts my day and my life.*"

> **!** What do you do with your d-supply bag while you swim or skate? I stop off at the lifeguard or manager's office, tell them that it's a diabetes supply bag, and say that I may stop by a few times for it during the day. It's more quickly accessible than leaving it in a locker, and in an emergency, you can tell staff to go to the office to retrieve your bag.

What I took away from the book is that I need to think about what caused a high or low blood sugar and see the reason behind it. This has changed my approach to sports, and now I don't go by the book—automatically giving her 15 grams of carbs before sports—but rather I tailor the number of carbs she has, whether or not to give her insulin up front, how often I need to check her blood sugar during the activity, and even if I need to do an extra blood sugar check eight to ten hours later, based on the individual sport and how Quinn's body reacts to it.

When Quinn starts a new class or has a new coach, I don't feel the need to fully train the staff because I know I will be there at the ready. I do, however, tell them that she has diabetes, that if she feels low she should come to me to test her blood sugar, and that if she begins acting unusual, passes out, or has a seizure, to have someone get me immediately. I tell them that she needs to be able to freely have breaks to get a drink of water or use the restroom, and that she may need a snack. Staying with her has never been a problem. One class she takes requires parents to leave the building, but I requested that we stay in the hallway, which worked out fine.

Since Quinn is in elementary school, one of us stays with her during all sports activities. Children who are in middle school and are more independent in their diabetes care might go to practices without a parent. Some preteens and teens text their parents to tell them their blood sugar during practices, or give a quick call. It's also important to have staff on hand who are knowledgeable in diabetes care, including the signs and symptoms of low blood sugar, treating hypoglycemia using the rule of 15s, and using glucagon. If the sport is associated with the school, then it will likely fall under the parameters of your child's 504 plan (see chapter 8) and they should make the necessary accommodations.

SPORTS MANAGEMENT

Ginger Vieira

Exercising with Type 1 diabetes is not easy at first. The balancing act with insulin, carbohydrates, and different types of exercise takes time to understand—but it can be done! As a parent, encouraging your children to be active early on in their life with diabetes is crucial. The obvious fear and most significant challenge in exercises with diabetes is hypoglycemia. On the other hand, you may have already witnessed tremendous spikes in your child's blood sugar during a soccer game or during sprints at a track event.

continued on next page.

SPORTS MANAGEMENT con't

Whether your child's blood sugar went low or went high during exercise, what you need to know is that there is a logical physiological reason as to why that happened. And most importantly, you need to know that there are absolutely things you could do to prevent those unwanted fluctuations.

The biggest thing you want to avoid is to purposefully let your child's blood sugar become high just to prevent hypoglycemia during exercise. While this may seem like the easiest approach, it isn't necessary and it is not healthy. Exercise while your body's blood sugar is high can not only prevent your muscles from performing at their potential, but it will also prevent weight-loss, put definite stress on your kidneys and can easily lead to DKA if your blood sugar continues to rise. Your goal is not to exercise with high blood sugars, but to maintain a blood sugar between 100 to 160 mg/dL during all types of exercise.

Let's break it all down:

Aerobic (or cardiovascular) exercise uses primarily glucose for fuel. That means that when your child is in basketball or soccer practice and their heart rates are consistently above 120 beats per minute for longer than 20 to 30 minutes, you can expect their blood sugar to drop.

The solution? If your child is using an insulin pump, you can reduce their basal rates during practice. If your child uses pens or syringes, they will need to prepare for their aerobic exercise by eating carbohydrates without taking insulin.

How much of a reduction should you program on their insulin pump? Everyone's needs are going to be different. Begin with a reduction of 50 percent during the practice itself and take good notes. By creating a "diabetes science experiment" around basketball practice, for example, you can eventually determine the best plan for that type of exercise.

How many carbohydrates should they consume? Again, everyone's needs are going to be different. I would suggest starting with 15 grams of carbohydrates for every 30 minutes of planned exercise to be on the safe side. By creating a "diabetes science experiment" around basketball practice, for example, you can track whether 15 grams of carbohydrates was sufficient for 60 minutes of practice, or if they need 30 grams.

Ginger's experience: As an avid athlete myself, I'm a big fan of hiking in Vermont. If I plan to go for a 2-hour hike up, and 1-hour hike down, I want to start my hike with a blood sugar between 100 – 160 mg/dL. At the start of the hike, I will consume approximately 25 grams of carbohydrates. After 45 minutes to an hour, I'll check my blood sugar and mostly likely find it to be around 120 mg/dL. Knowing that I have another hour of hiking uphill ahead of me, I will consume another 25 grams of carbohydrates.

At the top of the mountain, my blood sugar is 155 mg/dL. For me, that is ideal. I don't want to be higher than 160 mg/dL, but I also don't want to be near 100 mg/dL and dropping quickly either. Because I'm about to head downhill, which will not use nearly as much energy, I will consume maybe 5 to 10 grams of carbohydrates, or I will consume nothing and check my blood sugar again after 30 minutes of hiking downhill.

When your child's blood sugar rises during cardiovascular exercise:
If you find that an actual basketball game causes his/her blood sugar to rise due to the adrenaline and fun stress of competition while playing another team, you can and should adjust their insulin doses to help combat the temporary insulin resistance that is caused by those stress hormones.

Ginger's experience: As a competitive powerlifter, I learned quickly that the morning of competition day, my blood sugar would easily spike from 110 mg/dL to 280 mg/dL for no apparent reason, aside from the excited stress of competing. These competitions last all day long, so a quick dose of short-acting insulin wasn't going to help. Instead, I learned to increase my long-acting insulin dose the night before, sometimes by 25 percent,

continued on next page.

SPORTS MANAGEMENT con't

and that helped me keep a more stable blood sugar of under 180 mg/dL. It wasn't until my third competition that I actually had a full understanding and accurate plan for competition day.

If your child's blood sugar is too high or too low during or after basketball practice, then you know your next "diabetes science experiment" should include an adjustment based on your first experiment.

In anaerobic exercise (strength training, sprinting etc.) the body does not burn up glucose as quickly. In anaerobic exercise, your body is working at such an intensity, but for a much shorter duration before resting, that it cannot use oxygen for fuel as easily, and it does not use glucose in the same either. Instead, your body is actually breaking down muscle and releasing glycogen, which is then converted into glucose.

That means your child's blood sugar might actually rise during anaerobic exercise. If anaerobic exercise is combined with a higher-heart rate for a longer duration, such as circuit-training or jumping-rope, you may find that his/her blood sugar doesn't rise or drop.

Circuit-training and jumping-rope are both examples of exercise that involves high-intensity for several minutes, with a short period of rest before you begin again. In a pure aerobic or cardiovascular workout, there would be no rest period, leaving the heart-rate high continuously for a duration of 30 or more minutes.

The solution?

Your first step is to understand whether or not the type of exercise your child is performing truly is anaerobic. Something like football practice, while it may seem like a stop-and-go event, is likely to be more aerobic (cardio) in most cases, but some practices may actually be more anaerobic, depending on the drills performed!

Ginger's experience: When I am doing a 60-minute workout of jumping-rope and box jumps, my heart-rate feels as though it's through the roof the entire time; however, after each circuit of both exercises, I rest for at least two minutes, during which my heart rate drops. This makes this exercise far more anaerobic than aerobic. I could never sustain these exercises for a continuous duration of 30 minutes, let alone two minutes!

Through performing science experiments around this exercise, I've established that I can begin with my blood sugar in range, between 100 to 160 mg/dL, and not worry about it dropping. If I eat something at the start of the exercise, I cover it with insulin, or if I don't want food at that time, I do not eat anything. Because I am beginning with an in-range blood sugar, and there isn't any reason why my body would produce stress-induced hormones that might blunt my insulin sensitivity, my blood sugar stays exactly where it is.

In powerlifting training, however, I do notice a slight increase in my blood sugar. This is because the intensity of the anaerobic weightlifting causes a great deal of muscular breakdown, which causes the release of glycogen from my liver. This is not a bad thing, it simply means that glycogen is going to be converted into glucose and transported to those muscles that are being broken down. Without enough insulin, that glucose is actually going to sit in my bloodstream instead.

To prevent a high blood sugar during or after my training, I am always sure to consume a snack or small meal before training, accompanied by a full coverage of insulin for the carbohydrates in that meal. Because the spike I see in my blood sugar is usually only 30 to 50 mg/dL and I'm generally starting my training with a blood sugar under 160 mg/dL, I do not take extra insulin purely for that small spike.

In the end, it's all about creating experiments, taking good notes, and being patient as you continue to learn. Try to begin each experiment with an in-range blood sugar (100 to 160 mg/dL) so you can be sure you aren't adding extra variables to the experiment. Write down everything that is eaten before and during the exercise, the insulin taken, and the exact kind and length of exercise performed.

continued on next page.

SPORTS MANAGEMENT con't

Remember, there is always an explanation for a high or low blood sugar; if you don't know the explanation yet, that simply means you have more to learn!

Ginger Vieira has lived with Type 1 diabetes and celiac disease since 1999. Today she is a cognitive diabetes coach at Living-in-Progress.com, personal trainer, author, and freelance writer and video blogger. In 2011, Ginger published Your Diabetes Science Experiment. In 2009 and 2010, Ginger set 15 records in drug-free powerlifting with personal best lifts including a 308 lb. deadlift, 190 lb. bench press, and 265 lb. squat. She is the Mental Skills Coach for TeamWILD.org, and a diabetes health coach at DiabetesDaily.com. Find her YouTube Channel for diabetes video blogs at YouTube.com/user/GingerVieira.

Summer Fun

Amusement Parks

I love going to amusement parks in the summer. As a kid, I would ride the coasters over and over again. We have introduced our kids to the thrill of the amusement park, and they can't wait to go again. If you do a little planning ahead, you will have an enjoyable day. Visit the park's website and e-mail or call their guest services office to ask about specifics regarding accommodations that can be made for people with diabetes. I think you will find they want to be helpful, so you have a great experience. You may or may not need a letter from the doctor stating that the child has a medical condition and needs special accommodations.

Ask about passes for people with disabilities that allow you to jump to the front of lines or provide you with a time to return so that you aren't standing in lines. Sometimes these passes only work for the larger rides and coasters.

I suggest stopping by guest services after entering the park. They can give you a map with medical stations circled. You can obtain the medical accommodation pass for your family, and they can place a sticker on your supply bag that identifies it as containing medical supplies. Also, while many parks allow no outside food or drinks, a person with diabetes should be able to bring in snacks and drinks.

I like to pack a couple of water bottles that we can refill throughout the day to stay hydrated. Remember, there is a lot of blacktop at amusement parks, which turns up the heat! Pack enough food to cover regular snack times, plus a few extras in case you need them to recover from lows. I also pack a few extras for other family members. Applesauce pouches and organic fruit strips hold up well in a backpack or cooler. Food and drinks can be expensive at amusement parks, and you don't want to pay $3 or $4 for a snack to treat a blood sugar low. When you dine at parks, they probably won't have carb counts available. If you pull up The CalorieKing app on your phone (or toss the paperback in your backpack), you can make a good guess.

You may be wondering what to do with your diabetes supply bag when you are on the rides. On some rides, you can keep your bag with you, but for others it's not safe because it will obstruct seatbelts or could fly out of the car. There is usually a set of cubbies or a basket where you can put your supply bag while you're on a ride. We also had guest services put a sticker on our supply bag saying that it contained medical supplies. In case it was lost, it would be more likely to be returned to the office and reunited with us.

Blood sugar might also be on a rollercoaster while you are at amusement parks. Adrenaline can cause high blood sugar, but all that walking can cause lows! I suggest checking blood sugar regularly and being proactive. Staying hydrated and sticking somewhat closely to regular meal and snack times will also help. During our last amusement park trip, Quinn had a perfect 100 come up on the meter!

Water Parks

Considerations for water parks are similar to amusement parks, but I'm sure your first thought is how to keep everything dry. During our last visit to the water park, we

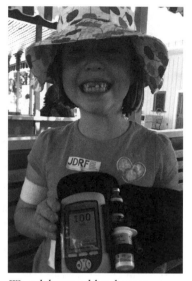

We celebrate a blood sugar reading of 100 by snapping a quick photo.

chose to stop at the first aid office and leave our d-supply bag with them, including a few snacks and juice boxes. We stopped by the office a couple of times during the day to check Quinn's blood sugar. Since the office was air-conditioned, we didn't have to worry about keeping insulin cool.

Since we left the supply bag, including our insulin, glucagon, and the remote for the insulin pump in the first aid office, I didn't

> **!** Rent a stroller for younger kids during park visits. Not only will kids be less tired and therefore less cranky, but you can cover more ground if you aren't dragging them along. Less walking means less chance of a blood sugar low. Plus you can throw your d-supply backpack in. We think it is well worth the $5 to $10 for the day for a double stroller.

want to feel completely helpless if Quinn's blood sugar plummeted. So, I purchased a waterproof pouch with a lanyard at our local camping store and used it to carry an extra meter, a few test strips, lancets, Smarties, and cake icing gel. I also gave my husband a small

> ! On extremely hot days, keep your insulin in your soft-sided cooler with your drinks and snacks. You could also use a Frio cooling pack if you aren't carrying a cooler.

waterproof box to keep in the pocket of his swim trunks that had cake icing gel and Smarties. While they do sell waterproof pouches that are touted as able to keep expensive electronics dry, I didn't want to risk getting the insulin pump remote wet.

Camping

Our family enjoys camping, and diabetes isn't going to stop us from getting outdoors and enjoying nature. We have a pop-up camper and tend to stay at state parks with electric hook-ups and shower houses. The things that make me the most uneasy about camping are having poor cell phone reception in case we need emergency assistance and being at least a half hour from the closest hospital. The reality is that we rarely have to make a call for medical assistance or need a hospital for diabetes-related care.

> ! Medical IDs are even more important when at amusment parks. If your child should become separated from you, staff will be able to call your cell phone if the number is engraved on the bracelet.

If you are concerned with being able to get medical assistance, there are two things you can do. Locate the accommodations for the camp "host." The host is a

> ! No food allowed? Even though there may be a rule at pools, water parks, and other venues such as sports arenas, against bringing anything in, they will allow you to bring in food and drinks for people with diabetes.

person or family who stays onsite throughout the camping season and can answer questions about the campgrounds. They often have a camper and a phone. You should also familiarize yourself with the ranger station. The rangers generally patrol campgrounds often and can be flagged down to ask questions or assist you.

The biggest issue while camping is keeping insulin cool. Our pop-up camper has a refrigerator, but if you are camping in a tent you need to keep it cool either by using a Frio cooling pouch or storing it in the cooler. If you use an ice-filled cooler, take care not to put the insulin directly on the ice. Instead, place the insulin in a plastic container and place that inside a plastic zipper storage bag. The air should keep it from freezing.

As with any type of travel, you need to pack enough supplies for the length of the trip. I usually take double what we need. The

> ! Most water parks have a centrally located first aid office. Ask to leave your d-supply bag there; not only will it be nice and dry, but the building is usually air conditioned.

campsite we normally go to is an hour from our house and 30 minutes from the nearest hospital and pharmacy. If we forget something, it wouldn't be too hard to get what we need. If you are camping or hiking in a remote area, pack more than you need; perhaps three times the normal supplies for that length of time.

Because our preparedness kit contains every diabetes supply

item we might need, I use that as our camping supply kit, making sure to refill it when we get back home. We also have a first aid kit in our camper. Since we camp frequently, I have a master packing list of all the things our family needs, including diabetes supplies. I keep a small food scale and a set of measuring cups in our camping gear to make carb counting easier.

We don't make any big changes in the food we take camping because of diabetes. To make carb counting easier, some foods can be portioned out ahead of time. I include plenty of fruit such as bananas, grapes, and cantaloupe, which I cut up ahead of time. We also eat a lot of peanut butter and jelly sandwiches with natural cheese puffs or chips as a side. I pack applesauce pouches and organic fruit strips to take while bike riding or hiking. I have a memory of my grandfather letting me get a box of Apple Jacks when he took me to the lake as a child. To carry on this tradition, I let my kids pick out a box of cereal—any kind they want—when we camp. We never buy sugary cereals at home, and this is a special tradition just for camping.

> ! Just because you are in the water doesn't mean your child doesn't need ID. Place a silicone bracelet that says "diabetic" on your child's wrist. There are also temporary tattoos that can be ordered online that say "diabetic" or "medical condition" and can be printed with information.

Plan ahead for the types of activities you might do while camping. We like to take our bikes with us, but biking around the state park usually sends Quinn's blood sugar low. I make sure to take a couple of juices and her supply bag with me when we ride. If you will be hiking for a long period of time, take not only your supply bag but extra snacks, lots of water, and low blood sugar treatments.

You will be thankful if the trail is longer than you thought it would be or you get lost. Always tell someone where you are going and take a buddy if possible. You can also carry walkie-talkies in case you need to communicate across the park.

When canoeing or boating, don't forget your supplies. I purchased a waterproof box which is big enough to hold an extra meter, glucagon, glucose tabs, a juice box, and snacks. But I don't put anything in it that I would be too upset about if it somehow ended up on the bottom of the lake! In other words, I don't put Quinn's insulin pump remote in the box. If she needs insulin, then we come ashore. I also have a rule that my kids always wear life jackets when they are near water. It doesn't matter if they are fishing off a dock or in a canoe, they must have one on.

S'MORES

Camping just isn't camping without making s'mores. You would be depriving your child of a life experience if you took them camping and didn't let them roast marshmallows over the campfire. S'mores are high in carbs, there's no getting around that, but blood sugar might not spike as high if they are eaten as part of a meal.

S'more
1 sheet of graham cracker = 11 carbs
1 marshmallow = 6 carbs
¼ Hershey chocolate bar = 6.5 carbs
Total = 23.5 carbs

Travel Time

Shortly after Quinn's diagnosis, we packed up the family for a last-minute trip by car halfway across the country on Thanksgiving to attend a funeral. One of the biggest challenges of traveling on Thanksgiving was finding a restaurant open at dinnertime! After this trip that took us from Illinois to Vermont to New Hampshire to Maine to Indianapolis and back home with an 18-month-old and a four-year-old, I knew we could tackle any road trip.

Quinn always wears her medical ID bracelet when she leaves the house, and when we travel I make double sure she has it on. When we were halfway home on our long car trip, my husband and I realized that we hadn't been putting it on her, because she was with us. But what if we were in a car accident and none of us could speak? The ID needs to speak for us. There are also window decals available online that state that the driver has diabetes or that a child on board has diabetes.

When traveling, I always pack three times the amount of supplies I think I will need, just in case. I also grab our preparedness kit since it has a backup of everything we could possibly need. I make sure to have contact numbers for our endocrinologist and pediatrician programmed into our phones, as well as the mobile apps of the major pharmacies in case we need something en route.

I like to stop every couple of hours when traveling with children to let them stretch their legs and go to the bathroom. Many rest areas have playgrounds. Blood sugar levels can rise when someone is sedentary in the car for long periods, and running around on the playground for ten minutes might help keep them even. Some diabetes educators recommend setting a temporary increased basal rate on insulin pumps during long periods of car or air

CAMPING WITH DIABETES

Excerpted from **Take a Hike—Tips and Tricks for Backpacking with Diabetes by Jen Hanson**

Growing up with type 1 diabetes (I was diagnosed in 1987 at the age of three) has, undoubtedly, provided some challenges when it comes to living life to the fullest out-of-doors, but these challenges have only made me stronger and led me to seek out greater adventures. I don't ever remember being afraid to camp, hike, or paddle with my diabetes. I don't recall ever resenting the trials life with diabetes brought on when it came to adventuring. If anything, I remember feeling more prepared, more organized, more in tune with my body because of my diabetes, and more ready to take on that next mountain peak, that next river bend, or that next backcountry bushwhack.

In 2009, I began working for Connected in Motion, a Canadian-based nonprofit organization that provides outdoor adventure and physical activity based experiential diabetes education opportunities for people with type 1. By 2010, we had set out on a cross-Canada tour with the hopes of meeting and engaging youth and young adults with type 1 diabetes in the outdoors— bringing them together to learn from one another and gain the skills to help each of them live life with diabetes to the fullest. We paddled, climbed, camped, and hiked our way from Canada East to Canada West. Following our adventures, which included a three-day adult canoe trip in Ontario, a five-day young adult hiking expedition in Whistler, BC, and a four-day adult hiking trip along the Juan de Fuca trail on Vancouver Island, we had time to reflect on the biggest diabetes challenges we faced and how we overcame them.

One of the trials I faced, repeatedly, during my two months on the trails was the nighttime low. During the first few days of any backpacking trip, when I'm working to get my insulin regime ironed out, I will inevitably experience a midnight low. But being prepared to treat a low, while huddled in a sleeping bag, in a tent, in the backcountry can be a bit tricky.

Among the outdoor community, it is a well-known fact that odors—be those from sunscreen, toothpaste, garbage, or food—attract wildlife. At Connected in Motion, we've heard stories, and even seen firsthand, the damage that can be caused by the animals we share the backcountry with when their noses lead them to the campsite of a forgetful (or ignorant) backpacker. A pre-pared backpacker, however, can significantly reduce the risk of an uninvited guest dropping in for a visit. Typically, all food, cosmetics, garbage and any other smell-emitting items are stored in bear lockers/bins or sealed and hung out of reach of wildlife. But this practice brings up an important question: Where do we keep supplies to treat nighttime lows?

Over the years, I have come across many peers—from recreational campers to bear safety experts and mountain guides—each with different experiences and opinions. I've toyed with different low treatments (my favorite for backcountry camping are glucose tabs), different storage locations (from a locked Pelican case in a location away from our sleeping area to a sealed Ziplock baggie stored inside my sleeping bag), and different low prevention strategies (dropping basal rates overnight, eating a larger pre-bed snack, setting alarms and checking through the night, or a combination of all of these).

In the end, my regime usually involves a carb- and protein-rich evening snack (like granola and peanut butter or a Luna bar), a reduced basal rate beginning up to two hours before I head to bed and a non-smelly, fast-acting source of glucose in a sealed container inside my sleeping bag. Despite being proactive in trying to prevent nighttime lows, the number of times I've had to break into my low stash for a nighttime fix certainly reaffirms my decision to keep carbs close by. A good friend and well-respected outdoor guru (and fellow type 1) once told me: "Keeping something such as a sealed granola bar on your person—inside your sleeping bag—to guard from lows is essential. There will be 50 other things that will be curious to a bear's nose before a sealed granola bar. Shoes, for example."

Jen Hanson has type 1 diabetes that was diagnosed when she was three. Since 2009, she has worked for Connected in Motion, a group that provides outdoor adventure and physical activities for individuals with type 1 diabetes (www.connectedinmotion.ca). The text is excerpted from an e-book Diabetes: Take a Hike—Tips and Tricks for Backpacking with Diabetes, which she cowrote with Chloe Steepe and Sarah Ketcheson.

travel to combat rises in blood sugar. Your diabetes educator or endocrinologist can make recommendations for your child.

I pack lots of snacks, including those already portioned out into easy 15-carb individual servings, as well as applesauce pouches. In the car, I usually bring a small cooler for water bottles and 2-carb drink pouches. I place the insulin in a plastic container and then into a zippered storage bag and place it at the top of the cooler, not inside the ice. You want to keep it cool, but not frozen. I also bring protein bars for bedtime snacks and a brick of juice boxes for treating lows.

When staying at hotels, ask for a refrigerator to store your insulin. These are provided at no extra cost for those needing them for medical reasons. When making your reservation, ask for the refrigerator ahead of time so they can assign you the appropriate room. If you are staying at a hotel because you are traveling to the endocrinologist or your child is staying at the hospital, ask if they can give a discounted hospital rate. When we were traveling almost 200 miles each way for our quarterly appointments, the hotel near the children's hospital provided us with a deep discount.

If you are traveling across multiple time zones, ask your care team how you should accommodate the change in schedule. Long-acting insulin needs to be taken every day within 30 minutes of the normal time. Basal rates on insulin pumps can be adjusted easily, and your diabetes educator or pump trainer can help you decide what changes to make, if any. If you are traveling across multiple time zones for an extended period of time, you will definitely need the assistance of your care team to make decisions about the timing of injections or basal rates, as well as eating schedules.

TRAVELING WITH DIABETES

Kelly Kunik

Traveling with diabetes is always interesting; at times incredibly frustrating, but always doable. It just takes some planning. Actually, it takes a lot of planning. But like I said, you can absolutely do it. My advice? Find out where you want to go, do some research on your destination, and book it! Then, make a list of absolutely everything you need to pack for your trip, including your diabetes supplies, and start packing.

The following items are just a few that I find really helpful when traveling with my diabetes:

- A note from your doctor stating that you or your child has diabetes and wears an insulin pump or uses syringes and is insulin dependant.
- Insulin
- Prescriptions in paper form. Also, if you use a national chain pharmacy, check to see if they have a branch near your destination just in case.
- Pump supplies/syringes
- At least three days supplies of extra pump supplies, syringes, insulin, and oral meds (if possible, I prefer a week's supplies).
- Glucose tabs
- Test strips
- An unopened vial of strips both in the carry-on and the checked luggage, so there is an extra, just in case.
- Lancets
- A box of granola bars and glucose tabs in the carry-on

And here are some tips to keep in mind:

- Don't rely on the airlines to provide you with food. They tend to run out by the time they reach the middle-numbered rows

continued on next page.

TRAVELING WITH DIABETES con't

and choices are extremely limited at best. Plus, the quality of food isn't terrific and prices are downright exorbitant!

• When flying and going through security checks, make sure to know your rights as a person and a person traveling with diabetes. Check the TSA website for details (www.tsa.gov). Be sure to check the website preflight because rules do change.

• I always ask for a visual inspection for my insulin pump and diabetes supplies when I first encounter a TSA security officer. According to TSA's website, you must request a visual "before the screening process begins." Requesting a visual inspection doesn't guarantee one so be prepared to stand your ground.

• Currently, the TSA offers "Disability Cards" to print out before you arrive at the airport. According to TSA rules, they won't prevent you from a pat down, but TSA says they may prevent a more intrusive one. I haven't tried the card yet myself.

So, now with your starting point regarding diabetes and travel—go book your trip and bon voyage!

Kelly Kunik is the creator of the blog, Diabetesaliciousness. She is a passionate diabetes advocate, speaker, writer, humorist and consultant. Kelly grew up in a family where four of eight family members (including herself, her father and two sisters) had type 1 diabetes.

CHAPTER EIGHT

School Days

For most families, sending a child with diabetes to school is one of the biggest challenges they face. After all, next to home, school is where kids spend the most time. You want them to be safe and well cared for, but also treated as similarly to the other children as possible. To ensure academic success, social happiness, and proper care, you will need to do some thorough planning and be actively involved; but, rest assured, it can be done.

Choosing a School

Choosing to send your child to a public or private school or keep him or her with you for homeschooling is a very personal decision that each family must make. There are pros and cons of each option relating to your child's diabetes.

Public Schools

Depending on your school district, you may or may not have a choice as to which school your child can attend. Often the school your child will go to is based on boundaries set by the district. Some districts, like the one we live in, allow the parents some choice based on criteria such as proximity to schools and demographics. These rules or guidelines may not be set in stone, and some accommodations might be made for children with a medical condition.

Why wouldn't you want to automatically attend the school that you are zoned for? Perhaps another school has a nurse on duty for more hours during the school day. Maybe there are children with diabetes already at the school, or even staff with diabetes. Maybe a school is closer to your office, allowing you to respond more quickly if you are needed. Or, the bus ride might be shorter to a different school. If you feel that a different school is in the best interest of your child, find out who can make decisions about school assignments and try to work with that person, stating your case. Discuss, don't demand … that never gets anyone anywhere!

Our district has "controlled" school of choice, meaning parents can make several ranked selections, and district uses a formula that takes into consideration proximity to schools, sibling priority, demographics, etc. During the selection process, my husband and I attended open houses at all of the schools we were interested in. While visiting, we asked key questions of the staff. I have to say that we had strong gut reactions at several schools, some of which surprised us.

The school that was closest to our home that we always thought we'd send our kids to was a definite no. Aside from the conditions of the school itself, which was dark and crowded, the assistant principal who gave us the tour told us that she rewarded the students with candy. I did not want to have an issue on my hands before school even started.

The school we favored had many positives, including a smaller size and lots of windows. As we toured the school, I told the assistant principal that our daughter has diabetes. His reaction was everything. While other schools told us they would learn how to deal with it, this assistant principal said, "We have a child with diabetes at the school already. We have experience and a system in place." His confidence was very reassuring. And since the school nurse was there only during lunchtime, he actually developed a strong relationship with Quinn because he did all of her blood sugar checks throughout the day and treated low blood sugars.

Once we made our selection, I attended a school board meeting about the school of choice program and introduced myself to the superintendent. I stated that I had a child with diabetes and that we had selected a particular school because there was already a child with diabetes there. It was also closest to both my husband's and my work so we could respond to any medical issues quickly. He instructed me to go through the process, and if we weren't happy with our assignment, he would make sure the appropriate staff would work with us on her placement. He stated that there is usually a seat or two that they can open up at each school for circumstances such as these. Luckily for us, we got the school we wanted.

An advantage of sending your child to public school is that public schools must comply with Section 504 of the Rehabilitation Act of 1973. An in-depth discussion of this can be found later in this chapter. Basically, public schools, by law, must make accommodations for your child with diabetes.

Private Schools

I'll admit that one of my first thoughts when my daughter was diagnosed was that we should consider a private school. However, as I researched, I realized this was not an option for us. First of all, tuition for private schooling is cost prohibitive for most families, ours included. Second, none of the private schools in our area have a nurse on staff, nor do they have to. However, the biggest sticking point—which is a big one—is that if the school is 100 percent privately funded, they do not have to make any special accommodations for your child.

I have seen many families hit a wall dealing with private schools that do not want to change policies or make exceptions for children with diabetes. Even private schools that do receive some public funds may be reluctant to make special accommodations. I really caution parents to weigh the pros and cons of private education when their child has a serious medical condition, because if they do run into issues, they may not have much recourse. That being said, if private education is something that your family feels strongly about, you can find ways to work with the school to meet your needs.

Homeschooling

Some parents decide to homeschool their child rather than go to a traditional school. If homeschooling wasn't already your plan before your child's diagnosis, really consider the pros and cons of keeping your child out of regular schools. Are you choosing homeschooling because it's a good fit for your family? Will you homeschool all of your kids? Would you homeschool if your child didn't have a medical condition? Are you choosing it because of fear of the unknown? Homeschooling is a great option for some families who can afford to have a parent leave the workforce, and those who have the fortitude and motivation to educate their children at home. Just keep in mind: the majority of children with diabetes go to traditional schools and do just fine there.

The 504 Plan

Section 504 of the Rehabilitation Act of 1973 is a federal law that ensures that those with disabilities, including diabetes, are not discriminated against. The law applies to all public schools, as well as private schools that receive federal funding. The law states that children with disabilities need to be given accommodations so that they receive an education comparable to that of other children who do not have disabilities.

The American Diabetes Association explains: "*The 504 Plan sets out an agreement to make sure the student with diabetes has the same access to education as other children. It is a tool that can be used to make sure that the student, the parents/guardians, and school personnel understand their responsibilities and work through challenges or misunderstandings to avoid problems in the future ... Section 504 applies to all public schools and to private schools that receive federal funds. The same plan would also be appropriate under another law that protects students with disabilities, the Americans with Disabilities Act (ADA). The ADA covers all public schools and all private schools except those run by religious institutions. (If the religious institution receives federal funds it is also covered.)*"

Putting the 504 in Place

Either before your child enrolls in school, or shortly after diagnosis if she or he is already in school, you will sit down with the school personnel who oversee 504 plans and begin the process. Typically, when a family requests a 504 plan for their child, a committee decides if the child should receive accommodations. In the case of diabetes, this first step is usually skipped and the 504 plan is automatically allowed.

While many families want the 504 plan in place the instant their child walks through the school doors, in reality it often takes months to get the plan in place. In fact, we chose to put guidelines for Quinn's care in place and not formalize her 504 plan until several months into the school year because we wanted to see what issues might arise that should be addressed in the document.

504 Plan Considerations

- Trained Diabetes Personnel: School will identify Trained Diabetes Personnel (TDP) who: 1) know how to test blood sugar levels and interpret the results; 2) know how to measure and administer insulin given by a syringe or insulin pump; 3) know how to respond to hypoglycemic events, including the use of the glucagon kit.
- Training: Training for TDP will be provided by a diabetes educator, nurse, or the parents.
- Location for Pre-Lunch Testing: School will provide an appropriate location for daily pre-lunch blood sugar testing and for lunchtime insulin by injection or pump.
- Access to Bathroom and Water: Child will be allowed unrestricted access to the bathroom, water fountain/or water bottle, snack, and the office when he or she is not feeling well. Child can carry water and extra glucose sources.
- Insulin Delivery: A TDP or nurse will supervise daily

glucose monitoring and administer insulin via injection or insulin pump. If a substitute is not aware of how to administer insulin, the school will call the parents.

- Testing: Glycemic conditions can have an effect on the child's testing, therefore: 1) blood sugar should be tested before important tests; 2) child needs to eat his or her regularly scheduled snacks even if they are during a test; 3) if diabetes-related activity (testing blood, snack, water, bathroom) must take place during a timed test, child will be given equivalent extension of time at the end of the test.
- Recognition of Hypoglycemic Conditions: All staff in charge of the child's class should have training or in-service on how to recognize hypoglycemic conditions.
- Fieldtrips: A TDP will accompany child on any trips away from school when a parent is unable to attend.
- Parental Notifications: Parents will be notified when food supplies need to be replenished, when the child has abnormal blood sugar and/or ketone readings, has insulin pump problems, when the schedule is significantly changed, or when the nurse is absent. Notification should occur as soon as possible.
- Substitute Teacher: Substitute teachers will be notified of child's diabetes and made aware of which staff members are TDP. Substitutes should be notified in the lesson plan that they are to use the TDP when needed.
- Lunch Time: Child can go to the front of the lunch line to get lunch and/or milk so that he or she has time to get food started before insulin is administered.
- Hallway Transportation When Hypo- or Hyperglycemic/

Not Feeling Well: Child must be accompanied by an adult
or responsible student when going to the office if he or she
is not feeling well.

- Emergency Supplies: Child's emergency supplies and
diabetes supply bag will be listed on the student roster to
insure they accompany the child during fire drills, field trips,
and any time he or she leaves the immediate school grounds.
- Lockdown Situations: Child will have blood sugar meter
and snacks in an additional location that is accessible
during a lockdown.
- Ketones: Child should use his or her blood ketone meter
(or urineketone strips) anytime that his or her blood sugar
is over 300.
- Attendance: Absences for diabetes-related medical appointments will not count against the child's attendance record.

Of course how your family manages your child's diabetes based
on the recommendations of your care team will dictate specific
wording and instructions. However, training staff, having access to
water and snacks, making sure that your child's supplies go with
her when she leaves the school grounds, making accommodations
for testing, and ensuring the child has enough time to eat lunch are
important points to consider. We didn't think about lockdown situations until another school in the district was on lockdown. Now
we have extra supplies in another location.

If your school has a full-time nurse in residence, then you may
have less need for more trained personnel. But the reality is that
many schools have only a part-time nurse, if they have one at all.

Some of these items may not seem important to your younger

child (like timed testing, which doesn't occur in our state until third grade). However, it is easier to add items when you first set up the 504 plan rather than try to add them later. Do note that a 504 plan is a fluid document, and you should be able to make changes at any time. If you have a change in care routine, such as changing from MDI to a pump, it is important to modify your 504.

More information on 504 Plans and sample plans can be found on the following websites:

- American Diabetes Association "Safe at School" www.diabetes.org/living-with-diabetes/parents-and-kids/ diabetes-care-at-school/written-care-plans/section-504-plan.html
- JDRF "Type 1 Diabetes in School" (including their School Advisory Kit) www.jdrf.org/index.cfm?page_id=103439
- Children With Diabetes (includes numerous sample plans) www.childrenwithdiabetes.com/504/

Training School Staff

When Quinn started kindergarten, we contacted the assistant principal during the summer to set up teacher training, and we have continued to do so every new school year. I like to call a meeting every year in the day or two before school starts to train all of the teachers who oversee her through-out the school day. This includes the classroom, art, music, and PE teachers, as well as the librarian, the assistant principal, and the

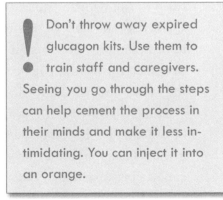

Don't throw away expired glucagon kits. Use them to train staff and caregivers. Seeing you go through the steps can help cement the process in their minds and make it less intimidating. You can inject it into an orange.

nurse. For some of these staff members, it is a refresher course; but for the classroom teacher, it is always brand new.

During the training session we go over key aspects of her 504 plan, especially the items that pertain to her daily school life, like access to water and the bathroom, checking blood sugar as needed, snacking at scheduled times, and checking blood sugar before important tests. I stress that her supply kit is listed as a separate child on the class roster, so that it is taken (and brought back) on fieldtrips, and any time she leaves the immediate school grounds, such as during a fire drill.

> ! ● If your child only requires a half dose of glucagon, write "mix all, inject half" on the outside of the plastic case.

I go over an instruction sheet I create for teachers line-by-line. It includes: the symptoms of low blood sugar; Quinn's usual symptoms and the language she uses to describe them; the rule of 15s; low blood sugar treatments; when to use glucagon and to call 911 if it's needed; and the symptoms of high blood sugar, along with protocol for checking and treating. I point out the three phone numbers they can call to reach my husband or myself, and encourage them to call with any questions. This sheet also includes a photo of Quinn so she can be easily identified, and it is placed in the lesson plan any time there is a substitute teacher. I put the instruction sheets in plastic page protectors and give one to each teacher, the nurse, and assistant principal.

I then show them the classroom kit, and we decide where each of the kits will be kept. We keep one in the classroom, usually on a shelf near the door, and one in the music room in the supply cabinet because that's where she would likely take shelter during severe weather or a lockdown situation. I go through the entire contents of the classroom kit because teachers might not be familiar with each of the items.

Although Quinn tests her own blood sugar, I show staff how to load a lancet, lance a finger, and apply blood to the test strip in the meter. If she were unable to think clearly or were shaky, someone might have to test her blood sugar for her. When I demonstrate, I'm always surprised at how much it hurts!

The training session culminates in a demonstration of the glucagon kit. I explain that, while the need for glucagon is not common, it is very important that if she is unconscious or having a seizure, the glucagon must be given immediately and 911 called. Not doing so can result in brain damage or death. This always scares teachers. I assure them it's like an insurance plan: you need to be prepared just in case, though you may never need it.

I think glucagon makes people nervous for three reasons. First, they are nervous because it's used in an emergency situation for the child, and they are afraid they won't remember what to do under pressure. Second, they are afraid that if they do it wrong they will do more harm than good. And third, that needle is really huge!

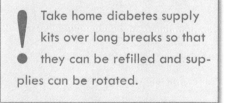

Take home diabetes supply kits over long breaks so that they can be refilled and supplies can be rotated.

When training school staff, I try to be as calm and reassuring as possible. I show them what the plastic case looks like and where they can find one in an emergency (in Quinn's d-supply bag, in the classroom kits, in the main office). I show them exactly how to use the kit and remind them to have someone call 911. After horrifying the teachers with the glucagon instruction, I assure them, once

STOCKING A DIABETES KIT FOR THE CLASSROOM

Stock all the supplies that your child might need during the school day. If the child may be in a different location during lockdown or severe weather situations, keep an extra supply kit in that room. I like to use soft-sided lunch boxes in bright colors, labeled with a medical alert sticker that includes the child's name, medical condition, and contact numbers.

Classroom Kit
- Blood glucose meter
- Test strips
- Lancing device
- Lancets
- Blood ketone meter (or urine ketone strips)
- Blood ketone strips
- Glucagon
- Glucose tablets
- Cake icing gel
- Smarties
- Snack
- Snack with protein*
- Bottled water*
- Instruction sheet

*In case of lockdown or severe weather situation.

Classroom Supplies
- Brick of juice boxes
- *The CalorieKing* book
- Small portable scale
- Alternate snacks

Supply Box for Office or Nurse's Station
- Supplies for two insulin pump changes
- Syringes
- Glucagon
- Blood glucose test strips
- Blood ketone test strips
- Batteries for pumps and meters
- Tape or adhesive
- Sharps container
- Insulin—stored in the office refrigerator (optional—may keep an extra vial of insulin at school if your child doesn't keep one in his or her supply bag.)

again, that they will get the hang of things even if they are feeling overwhelmed with the depth of information, and I tell them not to hesitate to reach out to the nurse, or assistant principal, or me with any questions.

After the regular staff leave, I stay a bit longer for more in-depth training with diabetes personnel listed on Quinn's 504 plan, which include the school nurse and assistant principal. With these staff I go into more detail about checking ketones and blood sugar, making sure she gets insulin for the food she actually eats at lunchtime, and how to use her insulin pump.

Communicating With Staff

I think it's extremely important to get off on the right foot with school staff. You want them to be in your corner and willing to help you because they will be taking care of your child for eight hours each day. I reiterate that they can call or e-mail me with any questions or concerns they might have, and I also check in with them from time to time to see if there are any issues or concerns.

As the parent of a child with diabetes, you hopefully received lots of training in diabetes management, but teachers and school staff receive only the minimal training you provide, so they are often overwhelmed and nervous. Try to make it as easy for them as possible and to make them feel more comfortable.

When problems arise, and it's likely you will encounter an issue at some point in your child's schooling, I feel the best results come from being level-headed, firm, and willing to discuss possible solutions. If it's a serious issue that can affect Quinn's health, I like to begin sentences with this phrase: "For Quinn's safety..." When an administrative decision was going to potentially affect Quinn's ac-

BUILDING A WORKING RELATIONSHIP WITH YOUR SCHOOL

Scott Benner

The relationship that you forge with your child's school is perhaps more important than the relationship you have with his or her endocrinologist. Sound crazy? Let me see if I can sway you ...

If your doctor is a bit gruff or hurries you in and out, that's not optimal, but you can always find a new endocrinologist. Changing the school your child attends is not so easy.

Depending on the age of your child at diagnosis, you could be looking at 13 years of schooling to navigate, and we want those years to be smooth ones. I've taken a long-term view of my relationship with my daughter Arden's school officials, nurses, and teachers. Even though we had a rough start, I kept my head, swallowed my pride a time or two, and focused on the more important long-term goal, opting to win the war and not every battle.

When I stopped in to chat with the principal at the end of the year prior to Arden starting kindergarten, I knew we were starting down a bumpy road. It was an informal meeting, meant to take the temperature of the folks that would be with Arden every day. This visit went well except for one almost innocuous moment: The principal laughed at me for showing up so many months before Arden would begin school. As I began to explain, I realized the principal didn't have the first idea of how challenging it would be to manage Arden's type 1 diabetes. She was basing what she knew on the much older and more mature type 1 children that had been through the school previously. This was the first time of many that I could have drawn a line in the sand and made my point that they "didn't understand." Instead, I gently expressed that Arden's management would be different than the other T1 kids at the school, and told her that I looked forward to speaking with her over the summer about Arden's 504 plan. I chose to plant a seed, take it slow, and see what I could get to grow.

I spent the next few months creating Arden's 504 plan, which is comprehensive without being bloated. It doesn't try to be fancy, and strives to be fair-minded, while covering all of Arden's needs. At our inaugural meeting, the school presented their own 504 plan—it was one page and consisted of five vague bullet points. When I saw it, I asserted myself for the first time saying, "I dare you to keep her alive for a week with that." However, you can't dig in your heels every time you disagree with something. It's more productive to think in terms of "How do I get this to where it needs to be?"

There are a number of reasons not to get emotional. The two most important ones are: 1) once you do, you look like an over-protective nut; and 2) they'll never take you seriously again if you do. Even though the person you are dealing with is a professional, people can have a very difficult time disconnecting themselves from their jobs and often take things personally. Your goal isn't to be correct; it's to get what you need for your child. In the pursuit of that goal you mustn't let the other side walk away feeling like you've beaten them or gotten something you didn't deserve; they need to feel good about what has transpired. You want the sight of your child to evoke caring and empathy, not the memory of you losing your cool in the principal's office.

The negotiation over Arden's initial 504 plan took four months, during which I had to educate our superintendent, as well as convey the importance of having school staff and bus drivers trained to recognize and react to type 1 situations. Along the way, there have been many opportunities for me to become angry, but I never did. I even smiled when one cafeteria employee said, "*I have a hard enough time dealing with the normal kids*" when I asked for carb counts.

A school aide once told Arden not to worry because "her OmniPod could be PhotoShopped out" of her school portrait. That comment

continued on next page

BUILDING A WORKING RELATIONSHIP WITH YOUR SCHOOL con't

made me crazy, but instead of entering into a situation that would have only served to dismantle the relationship that I've built, I called the school and explained why it wasn't optimal to give Arden the impression that she should be ashamed of the device that keeps her alive. The staff was properly sorry for what had transpired, and in all honesty, the person that said it wasn't being nasty, she just wasn't thinking. So, when they started to apologize, I wouldn't let them; instead, I apologized for the uncomfortable moment, and simply reinforced that this wasn't the message we should be sending.

In the end, this isn't about being right. It's about the players in the situation feeling empowered to help my daughter live her life as normally and as healthy as possible. It's about being able to ask for a favor without it feeling like a favor. It's about getting what I need for Arden as easily and as completely as I can.

Today, there is probably nothing I could ask for that wouldn't be handled with a smile, because I have developed a personal relationship with each person I deal with at the school—relationships that were grown one seed at a time.

I've been a full-time parent for more than twelve years (the last six

cess to care by trained personnel at school, I wrote a letter to the president of the school board and laid out each of my reasons beginning with "For Quinn's safety ..." The reality is that administration often looks at risk assessment and the bottom line when making decisions, and if it's an issue with potentially severe consequences, particularly to a child's health, they may reconsider. Hopefully, you can resolve issues before pulling out this big gun.

In general, I think school staff wants to be helpful and give your child the diabetes care she or he needs. But if you have issues that can't be resolved, you can always go up the chain of command. As a last resort, you may need to enlist the help of outside entities such of them with a type 1 diabetes child), so I understand the challenges and joys of this role. Though our numbers are growing, I am still in the minority being a man in this position. I'm still a guy (hey, I love sports!), but I'm also not embarrassed to carry a pink purse when Arden gets tired of holding it. As a matter of fact, none of what I do has ever made me feel embarrassed. I'm a full-time parent, and I'm proud of the things that I spend my days doing.

So, if I may be so bold, I have a message for the lionesses of the type 1 diabetes community. I know from watching my amazing wife how powerful a mother's love can be. When a mother's instincts kick in, I certainly wouldn't get in between you and your child's well-being. But sometimes, you have to suppress your natural instincts in favor of the long-term goal.

Scott Benner has been a stay-at- home father since 2000. As a diabetes advocate and social media author Scott shares his daughter's life with type 1 diabetes from his perspective on his website, www.ardensday.com. Scott's writing is honest, transparent, and a great resource for parents of, as well as people with, type 1 diabetes.

as the American Diabetes Association, a group well versed in the rights of students at school.

The School Nurse

Hopefully, your school has a nurse, but many school districts don't have the funding to place full-time nurses in every school. Some have part-time nurses who visit several schools, while others have only one nurse to oversee all students in the district or no nurse at all.

In the three years that Quinn has been in school, we have had a range of nursing scenarios, and we've done our best to make each

TIPS FOR NAVIGATING THE SCHOOL DAY

Lunch Time

- Kids have a very short period of time to eat their lunch. Children with diabetes should be allowed to go to the front of the line to get their meal or milk.
- Ask if your school district publishes their menu and nutritional data on their website.
- If you need a substitution, ask for it. We ask that Quinn be given fresh fruit instead of juice when it's served because juice can spike her blood sugar. The school district might require a letter from your doctor.
- Ask that the nurse not hover over your child, as socialization with peers is an important aspect of school.
- Ask that injections or insulin by pump be given promptly so that your child doesn't miss recess, which is also important for socialization and daily physical activity.

Substitute Teachers

- Lesson plans should clearly identify that your child has diabetes and specify who is trained in your child's diabetes management.
- Include a simple one-to-two page instruction sheet including symptoms and treatments for low blood sugar. This instruction sheet should have a photograph of your child so a substitute teacher can identify her.
- The daily schedule should include times that diabetes-related activities ought to occur, including scheduled blood sugar checks and snacks.
- Remind the substitute teacher that the child has free access to water and the bathroom, and may need to see the nurse or other staff throughout the day.

Lockdowns and Severe Weather

- Lockdowns and severe weather are hopefully uncommon, but you need to develop a plan.
- Place an extra supply kit in the room where your child is likely to be during a lockdown or when students take cover for severe weather.
- Stock the supply kit with a blood glucose meter and test strips, fast-acting sugar for treating low blood sugar, glucagon, and snacks and water in case they are there for a long time. The kit should include a simple one-to two page instruction sheet

including symptoms and treatments for low blood sugar and your phone number.

- Develop an exit strategy. Is there a window or another way for emergency workers to get to your child in case of a severe hypoglycemic event?

- Decide on a form of communication between the teacher and emergency workers or administration. Does the teacher have a cell phone, is there an intercom system, or can they be given walkie-talkies?

Taking the Bus

- Ask if your child can be the last one picked up in the morning and the first one dropped off after school. This will shorten the amount of time your child spends on the bus.

- Have your child's blood sugar tested at the end of the school day before she or he gets on the bus. Work out a plan to treat low blood sugar on the bus. It may include having the child eat a snack, notifying the bus driver or monitor, and/or calling you.

- Is there a bus monitor? The monitor and the bus driver should be trained, just like school staff,

to identify and treat low blood sugar.

- Have your child ride with a sibling or a buddy who can let the bus driver or monitor know if your child is having a low blood sugar, and can also make sure that your child gets home safely each day when dropped off at the bus stop.

Fieldtrips

- A trained person, besides the teacher, should accompany your child on fieldtrips. This can be the nurse, if available.

- The teacher may be too busy keeping track of the other students. A designated person, such as the nurse or yourself, can make sure blood sugar is checked and snacks are given at the scheduled times, and can treat low blood sugar.

- If the nurse is not available, consider volunteering as a chaperone.

- Don't forget the diabetes supply bag. List it as a student on the roster so that it is accounted for before leaving school grounds and is not left behind.

one work. In kindergarten, the nurse was there for the last half of lunch only. The assistant principal cared for her during other times of the school day, including checking her blood sugar before lunch. Then, a nurse was hired to float between several schools, but was stationed at our school. She was there for the entire lunch period, and was able to check on Quinn mid-morning and then again in the afternoon before she left. This nurse was a gem. She truly loved Quinn and was very communicative with me, which made me confident in her ability to take care of my child and make decisions. When she told us during this school year that she was leaving the district, I cried.

Developing good relationships with the staff members who care for your child is important not only for your child's well-being and safety, but also for your peace of mind. Although school nurses are trained in basic care, you are the person who knows your child's diabetes the best. You should try to form a friendly relationship with the nurse, while at the same time ensuring your child is cared for in the manner you think is appropriate. The school nurse can be your child's best advocate during the school day, and should get to know your child so as to be able to detect when your child is experiencing low or high blood sugar.

What if your school doesn't have a nurse? Laws on who can administer insulin vary by state, and individual school districts may have their own set of guidelines. Ideally, if there is no nurse, there are other school personnel who can be trained in your child's care. The American Diabetes Association has a list of laws and policies by state (www.diabetes.org/living-with-diabetes/parents-and-kids/diabetes-care-at-school/legal-protections/state-laws-and-policies.html), which can help inform you as to the type of diabetes management you should expect from your school, and from whom.

If your school has no nurse and your state prohibits non-medical staff from administering insulin, you are stuck between a rock and a hard place. Many parents facing this situation must visit school each day to give their child insulin at lunchtime. Some parents are forced to leave the workforce to be on call during the school day. In my opinion, this is an injustice because parents shouldn't have to choose between being employed and keeping their child safe at school.

Recently Suzanne Elder, a parent in Illinois who was forced to leave her job to care for her child during the school day, brought about new legislation to improve this type of situation for other families. *The Care of Students with Diabetes Act* allows non-medical staff to be trained to care for children with diabetes at school, and provides protection for these employees, as well as spelling out a number of other stipulations to help make children safe at school. This act is a model for parents in other states that do not have such provisions afforded to their children.

> **!** Work with your child's teacher and nurse to find the best time of day for special birthday snacks, so your child can be included and not sit there with an empty plate or boring alternative snack while other kids enjoy cupcakes. Special snacks might be given right after lunch so the nurse can give insulin, or at the end of the school day so you can bolus when you pick his or her up.

Talking to Other Students

There are two camps when it comes to educating classmates about diabetes. Some parents want to educate all of their child's classmates about diabetes. For younger grades you can easily educate children by having a short show-and-tell, including reading an age-appropriate book about diabetes. Tell children in simple terms what diabetes is (that your child's pancreas does not work and she can't make her own insulin), and that they won't catch it, which might be a common fear of young children. Show them your child's blood glucose meter and supply bag, and explain that they may see your child checking blood sugar or even getting an injection, but this shouldn't worry them. Tell them that your child might have to eat extra snacks, like on the way to PE, or that she may have to have juice if her blood sugar is low. Instruct them that if they ever notice your child acting differently, or if they can't wake her up, to let a grown-up know.

> ! • Volunteer to bake the cookies or cupcakes for class parties. There will probably be treats at parties, and if you make them yourself, at least you'll know the carb count.

The other camp doesn't want to bring even more attention to their child, thus making the other children think he or she is different right out of the starting gate. We chose this approach for several reasons. While we made sure that teachers and staff were educated and trained, we decided not to do formal teaching to the children. Instead, we took a "wait and see" approach. We found that children asked Quinn, the teacher, and the nurse questions as they had them, and that Quinn was confident enough in herself to respond. On many occasions when I was at the school, children would ask me

> ! • Have an alternate treat available just in case the special snack is completely inappropriate.

specific questions like how Quinn got diabetes, why she has to check her finger, and why she had to get shots.

In kindergarten, Quinn took it upon herself to do a show-and-tell. She displayed her medical ID bracelet, told the kids about checking her blood sugar and getting insulin, and fielded questions. I was proud of her for taking the initiative when she was ready to educate her peers. I wish I had been a fly on the wall that day!

And Then There Are the Parties

You've tackled all the logistics of 504 plans, training nurses, and making sure your child is safe at school—and now you have to deal with parties, which present their own set of challenges.

Quinn's kindergarten teacher advised parents that birthday snacks should have about 15 carbs, provided a list of possible treats, and said she needed advance notification. Unfortunately, that rarely happened. In fact, I often saw parents walking into school with a tray of gigantic cupcakes. At the time, Quinn was still on injections, and the nurse was only there for 15 minutes. The only way she could have participated was for me to leave work, which I wasn't going to do on a weekly basis! The teacher and I decided to keep a stash of Oreo Cakesters for Quinn to have when guidelines weren't met. Quinn actually thought this snack was great. Later, I began bringing the mega-carb birthday treats home for her to have with a meal.

In first grade, the nurse was there more often, so the teachers, nurse, and I decided that birthday snacks would be given right after lunch, and the nurse would estimate the carbs and bolus with her insulin pump. This system worked well for everyone. In second grade, we decided that birthday treats would be given at the end

TAILS OF LOVE: LIFE WITH A DIABETIC ALERT DOG

When the bell chimes, over 600 students spill into the hallways of Pioneer Middle School and make their way to lockers and classrooms. This is Charlie's favorite part of the school day. It gives him a chance to stretch his legs—all four of them. The kids aren't allowed to pet him, but many wave or say "hey, Charlie" as the big, caramel-colored standard poodle pads along the corridor. He acknowledges their greetings with a wag of his tail, but his focus remains on the girl walking next to him—Tori, a bright, active 11-year old who has type 1 diabetes.

Charlie is a diabetic alert dog, and he takes his job seriously. Once they arrive at Tori's next class, he lies quietly at her feet, where he stays, unless he detects a change in her blood glucose level. He may not be interested in seventh-grade science, but human biology is his specialty. If Tori experiences high or low blood sugar, her body releases chemicals that change the scent of secretions it produces. Though usually unnoticeable to the human nose, these changes are easily detected by Charlie's superior sense of smell and his training.

"I typically have lows around second hour and before sixth hour," says Tori. "Charlie alerts me by putting his paw on me. If I don't pay attention, he keeps bugging me, and if we're at home, he'll bark at me. Then he sits in front of me and watches attentively to make sure I test myself and have a snack or take insulin."

Tori Row was diagnosed with type 1 diabetes when she was two years old. Her mother, Kathy, recalls that she never slept well. During the day, she was a finicky eater and seemed unsettled. But no one suspected diabetes. Then, one day in 2002, she became very ill, and a routine urine test revealed a dangerously high sugar level. After a five-day stay at the University of Michigan Children's Hospital, the Row family took their daughter home, overwhelmed and anxious. It was the first time since her birth that Tori slept through the night, but for her parents, sleepless nights would become the norm.

Even as they adjusted to Tori's diagnosis and got into a routine, worry lurked in the background like a shadow. Many parents of children with this medical condition will attest that it feels like you can never stop thinking about them, especially through the night. It was during one of these restless nights that the family dog, which was not a trained alert dog, came into Kathy's bedroom and began pawing at her. The dog led Kathy into Tori's room, where she became very agitated and would not leave her side. When Kathy tested her daughter, she found that her blood sugar was very low. That experience prompted the family to begin researching diabetic alert dogs.

"We still do all the same things we used to—regular testing, injections and snacks," says Kathy. "But with Charlie, we have an added level of security. He gives us peace of mind, and is a wonderful companion for Tori. And, he's proved himself many times. One night, during a sleepover, he started nudging all the girls, and when that didn't work, he came and barked at me. When I tested Tori, her sugar was 75."

Studies show that alert dogs are amazingly accurate at detecting high and low blood sugar. In fact, Kathy notes that Charlie will often alert Tori when her blood sugar is starting to fall. It may be normal when she tests, but he senses that it is beginning to drop before she experiences symptoms. Charlie also alerts to rising blood sugar, which may help her lower her A1c and avoid complications over the long-term. Diabetic alert dogs can help older children become more independent, and give adults more freedom.

Alert dogs receive extensive training in both obedience and blood sugar detection, and that training continues at home using a sock or other clothing item when the person's sugar is low or high, or sometimes a cotton ball coated with saliva. While there are many organizations that train and offer alert dogs, the Row family warns those who are interested to do their homework and carefully research the facility. With a price tag of $6,000 to $8,000, on average, as well as a significant time commitment and the strong emotional bond that forms, you want to make sure the organization has a good reputation for training and follow-up. It goes without saying; the family should also be dog lovers.

Charlie goes everywhere with Tori, except dance class (too distracting!),

continued on next page

TAILS OF LOVE: LIFE WITH A DIABETIC ALERT DOG con't

and the family even travels with him. His vest identifies him as a service dog and gives him access to public places. But, when the vest comes off, look out: Charlie knows when he's off duty.

"He starts running around like crazy and playing with our other dogs," notes Tori, while affectionately rubbing Charlie's soft, curly head, which is lying on her lap. "He does get in trouble sometimes, but we love him. We treat him like a pet at home." From the look in his big brown eyes, the love is mutual.

What advice would Tori give a family considering a diabetic alert dog? "Get one, if you're up for it. He is a lot of work, but he's definitely worth it."

The Row family lives in Canton, Michigan with their three dogs, including Charlie, a diabetic alert dog. Their daughter, Tori, was diagnosed with type 1 at age two. She is now an active preteen who attends middle school with Charlie, and loves to dance.

of the school day, and I would bolus for them at pick up. My point is that you need to work with the teachers and nurse to develop a plan so that your child can participate as fully as possible in birthday celebrations.

In addition to birthdays, schools often celebrate Halloween, the December holidays, and Valentine's Day, which probably involve sweet treats. For me, the best way to deal with these events is to volunteer. You can volunteer in two ways that will help your child participate fully in the celebration.

First, volunteer to coordinate the menu or at least bring some of the food. I'm the room parent for Quinn's class, so I get to make the sign-up sheet for party food. At one of the recent parties, the list included carrots, grapes, cheese, drinks, and mini cupcakes— and I signed up to make the cupcakes! By making the treat myself, I know the exact number of carbs so there is no guessing game.

Second, you can volunteer to help in the classroom with the party. When I am at the parties, I can watch how much my daughter eats and give her an appropriate bolus. Even if there is a school nurse, you can probably estimate the carbs and give the bolus a little more unobtrusively than a nurse could.

CHAPTER NINE

Rx for Sick Days

It's unfortunate that the minor illnesses that keep most kids home from school for a day or two can send our children with diabetes to the emergency room. Illness can cause blood sugar to run high or low, depending on the ailment and the way your child's body reacts. That means our type 1 kids need a little extra TLC when they're sick, including more frequent blood sugar checks. But don't panic: by arming yourself with some information and planning ahead, you will be able to manage sick days with more peace of mind.

Sniffles, Stuffy Noses, and Allergies

Colds and other viruses, while annoying to everyone who gets them, could have an additional side effect on type 1 kids. When the body fights an illness, blood sugar might run higher as part of the immune system's response. Allergies can also have the same effect. In addition to elevated blood sugar from the body's fight against the virus or allergen, medications used to treat these conditions might also raise blood sugar.

Sometime after Quinn's diagnosis, when she was on an antibiotic that came in a huge bottle, I realized there might be a lot of carbs in over-the-counter and pre-scription medicines. I asked the pharmacist if he knew the carb count (he didn't), and of course, the bottle didn't have any information. It makes me wonder why medications aren't required to list nutritional information like food items do. It would *really* be helpful.

> ! A list of the carbohydrate content of some children's medications can be found on the Pediatric Care Online website. www.pediatriccareonline.org/pco/ub/view/Pediatric-Drug-Lookup/153888/0/carbohydrate_content_of_medications

The pharmacist advised me that if there is a pill or tablet option, it will likely have less sugar than the liquid form. For instance, the children's chewable acetaminophen contains less sugar than the liquid suspension formula. I began reading labels, and I've noticed that some children's medications are made with artificial sweeteners, while others use sucrose (sugar). There is also a big difference between chewable vitamins and the gummy ones. Vitamins usually do carry a nutrition label, which includes the serving size and carb count.

As with many aspects of diabetes care, the way your child's blood sugar reacts to a cold or allergies may differ from the experience another child has—and it may vary from one cold to another. The only way to be sure is to check blood sugar more frequently and adjust accordingly. Also, don't be afraid to call your care team if you're having trouble keeping blood sugar in range.

Infections

Illnesses such as strep throat, ear infections, and respiratory flu tend to affect blood sugar more than colds and allergies. As mentioned, blood sugar often rises as the body fights off an illness, and the body has to work hard to ward off an infection. Several

> ! Medications that contain acetaminophen can interfere with the readings on the DexCom continuous glucose monitor because they change the reaction of the sensor in the interstitial fluid.

times I have seen Quinn's blood sugar run high for several days in a row for no apparent reason. Readings hover in the 200s, and correction after correction doesn't seem to bring them down. I have learned through experience that these blood sugar spikes are often a red flag of impending illness.

I try to be proactive when she does get sick, not only because illnesses wreak havoc on her blood sugar, but also because I don't want the illness to drag out or cause complications that require even more care. When the H1N1 flu strain was first being diagnosed around the country, she exhibited some of the symptoms of both strep throat and the flu. I got her into pediatrics right away, where they did a throat swab for the strep and a nasal swab for the flu. Because diabetes puts her at a higher risk for complications, the doctor chose to treat her immediately. The medication oseltamivir, sold under the name Tamiflu, can be given to people within the first two days of symptoms of respiratory flu. It stops the

> ! Steroids used to treat some conditions can raise blood sugar. If your child needs to use a steroid, ask your endocrinologist how this might affect his or her diabetes.

spread of the virus in the body and can shorten the duration of symptoms.

Stomach Bugs

If there is one illness that makes parents of children with diabetes frantic, it's the "stomach flu" or, more precisely, gastroenteritis (which is really not a form of flu at all, but inflammation of the stomach and intestines caused by a virus, bacteria, or parasite). Because gastroenteritis is not caused by the influenza virus, which causes respiratory flu, it cannot be vaccinated against. It can hit anyone, at any time, without warning, and there's no stopping its effects. Stomach bugs usually run their course in a day or two in healthy people, and may keep children home from school. But in people with diabetes, it can quickly turn from bad to worse, which is why we need to be on our A-game.

Why is a stomach bug so bad for kids with diabetes? Because vomiting affects blood sugar and dehydration can cause ketones, and possibly DKA. We have dealt with stomach bugs twice since Quinn's diagnosis. The first time she threw up, I checked her blood sugar, and it was in the 300s. A check of her urine revealed she was

> ! Ask your endocrinologist what cold and cough medications can be recommended and then keep a supply on-hand for those middle-of-the-night sniffles.

developing ketones. At that time, we were still doing injections. An extra bolus didn't bring her blood sugar down, nor reduce the ketones, and we ended up taking her to the ER on the advice of the endocrinology office. The second time it happened she had just eaten her bedtime snack and gotten insulin to cover it. She vomited up her snack, but still had that active insulin in her system, so her blood sugar remained low. She couldn't keep down juice, and reducing, and eventually suspending, her basal insulin with her insulin pump did nothing to bring her blood sugar back in range. She was developing ketones. At 2:00 AM, the endocrinologist on call told me to take her to the ER for an IV drip of fluids to hydrate her, dextrose to get her blood sugar back up, and anti-nausea medications to stop the vomiting.

There are two at-home courses of action you and your doctor can discuss that may keep you out of the ER. I find that communication with the endocrinology office, even if it means awakening the on-call physician in the middle of the night, is the key to dealing with stomach issues. They can help talk you through steps that might get it under control at home, or tell you when it's time to jump in the car and seek medical treatment.

The first course of action may be the anti-nausea medication called ondansetron, sold under the name Zofran, which can stop the vomiting. Some endocrinologists will prescribe this and allow families to keep it on hand, just in case. However, some endocrinologists will not prescribe it in advance because vomiting is also a sign of appendicitis, which the medical staff wants to rule out. The doctor may call in a prescription for Zofran, or direct you to the ER to receive it.

If blood sugar is low and children can't ingest and keep down fast-acting sugar with a stomach bug, a technique referred to as "mini-glucagon" might be suggested by your endocrinologist. An explanation of this technique is given in the book *Understanding Diabetes* (the Pink Panther book). Glucagon is mixed, and a small dose is given using a regular insulin syringe. The dosage is determined based on the age of the child. Ask your endocrinologist about this technique and the proper dosage for your child, as it has helped many parents manage stomach bugs at home without a trip to the ER.

Checking Ketones

In chapter 4, I described the two methods of checking ketones—using urine ketone test strips or using blood ketone test strips. I'm a big proponent of blood ketone strips because they are easy to use, even in the middle of the night on a sleeping child, and because they give real-time results. It was drilled into us during our education at diagnosis that we need to check ketones when blood sugar is extremely high. It was emphasized again when we began using the insulin pump—always check ketones when blood sugar is very high in case insulin is not being delivered.

What I didn't realize is that ketones can also develop with low blood sugar. This seems counterintuitive based on all that I have read and learned about diabetes. Vomiting can cause the development of ketones even in people who don't have diabetes. During our last battle with gastroenteritis, Quinn's blood sugar was low, and yet she was developing ketones.

To get rid of ketones you need a combination of insulin, carbs, and fluids. Your endocrinologist can help you decide how to take action to reduce ketones depending on the type of illness your child has, and whether or not he or she can keep down foods.

Cuts and Scrapes

When Quinn was diagnosed, I remember being told during our training that she shouldn't run around outside without her shoes on. I think that particular freedom—frolicking outside barefoot, jumping through sprinklers, and feeling the soft grass beneath her feet— was one of the losses I was most saddened about, especially because she spent so much time playing in the backyard and helping me in the garden. I bought her several pairs of flip-flops to slip on as she headed out the back door each day. I was so thankful when I double checked with our endocrinologist later on, and she told us we could lift this ban so long as she didn't have open cuts or sores on her feet,

> If your child will be in the hospital for an extended period of time, update family and friends with a free Caring Bridge page at www.caringbridge.org

and she wasn't playing in an area where she might step on a nail or some other sharp object.

The problem is that people with neuropathy, or loss of feeling in their feet, might not realize they have cut their foot and could get a nasty infection if a cut isn't properly cleaned and tended to. The reality is that in people with diabetes, cuts and scrapes might heal more slowly, increasing the possibility of infection. Common sense treatment of these minor injuries is to clean the wound, apply antibiotic cream or ointment, keep it covered so it can heal, and watch it carefully.

When to Go to the ER

I'm big on communicating with medical staff during times of illness to get guidance. Sometimes I find myself calling both our local pediatrician, who can help guide us on the illness itself, and the endocrinologist, who can help us deal with the diabetes aspect. The pediatrician and endocrinologist can give recommendations, which may include prescribing the anti-nausea medication and/or giving mini-glucagon, as described above, and pushing fluids when appropriate.

Sometimes no matter what you do, you just can't manage the illness and the diabetes together, and it's time to go to the ER. When that happens, make sure your endocrinologist calls the emergency room before you arrive. If possible, head to an emergency room that has a pediatric endocrinologist on staff.

I cringe when I think of the bill that arrives along with a visit to the ER, but when it comes to getting my daughter medical care when she needs it, the price of an ER visit seems small in comparison to keeping her healthy and complication free. Your medical team may suggest checking into the ER for anti-nausea meds to stop vomiting, fluids to treat dehydration and flush ketones out, and either extra insulin to bring high blood sugar down or a dextrose drip to get low blood sugar up, under the care of the medical team at the hospital.

If you find yourself going to the ER for nondiabetes-related emergencies, such as a broken bone or stitches, be sure to let the medical staff—from the triage nurse to the ER doctor—know that your child has type 1 diabetes.

SICK DAY SNACKS

When battling illness at home, whether strep throat or a stomach bug, your child may need to "drink her carbs," so she can receive some insulin to keep blood sugar in range and ketones in check. It's a good idea to keep a few of these stocked at home for sick days.

Liquid Snacks

Popsicles (not sugar-free)	Apple juice
Gatorade or other sports drinks	Regular Sprite or 7-Up (not diet)
Pedialyte	Regular JELL-O (not sugar-free)
Soup (clear broths)	

When they are ready for something more substantial, these solid foods are often gentle on the tummy and tasty.

Solid Foods

Saltine crackers	Applesauce
Vanilla wafers	Ice cream or frozen yogurt
Graham crackers	Pudding
Dry toast	Sherbet or sorbet

UNDERSTANDING FLU, THE FLU SHOT, AND THE PIRATES OF THE CARIBBEAN

Wil Dubois

The doctor wants your kid to get a flu shot. Every year. Why? And why every year?

I'll tell you. But first we have to talk about pirates, because flu viruses are like the pirates of the Caribbean. You see, flu reproduces by taking over other cells, hijacking them in an act of biological piracy. Oh, and I'm not talking about Disney Johnny Depp–type pirates here. I'm talking about the ship-sinking, thieving, plundering, skin-you-alive-and-feed-you-to-the-sharks kind of pirates of the olden days. I think we can all agree we don't want any of those in our bodies.

So how does one go about eliminating pirates? Well, you send the Royal Navy out after them, of course, in the guise of your immune system. But the problem is that there are a lot of different kinds of pirates. Oh, and lots of other ships out there that may or may not be harmless. *Were those pirates, or just scruffy-looking merchant seamen with a shipload of bamboo from Bangkok?*

Just how many different flu pirates are there for your immune system to learn about? There could be as many as 1,000,000 strains of flu. Oops. Now there are 1,000,001. They evolve that fast. So the Royal Navy needs some anti-pirate warfare training.

And that's what a flu shot is. It's a way of priming the pump, helping train the immune system to recognize pirates so they can, you know, kill them on sight.

A traditional syringe-and-needle flu shot is just a bunch of dead pirates floating in sea water. It's an inactivated vaccine, a killed sample of the very real pirates that are out there planning winter mischief. It's a safe way to introduce your body to a new threat; your immune system can study the enemy and learn how to defeat it with no risk of getting sick. It's like taking the Royal Navy Marines down to the dock-side morgue to see some real pirate bodies to help them recognize live ones out on the open sea.

Another way to teach the immune system to deal with invaders is to give it a small amount of living virus that has been very much weakened. The nasal snort type of flu shot is an example. Think of them as pirates who've had the crap kicked out of them by Royal Marines. Not dead yet, but kicked to the brink of death. They're in no shape to put up much of a fight, much less steal ships. Medically, we call them live attenuated vaccines.

Which kind should you get your kiddo? Well ... that's not as simple a question as it sounds, so chat with your doc about the best choices for your crew.

Why a new shot every year? Isn't last year's still on the job? Sure. But remember what I told you about the number of strains of flu, which has now jumped to 1,000,054 while you've been reading this? Right. Every year the flu is, well, not last year's flu.

So how *well* does the flu shot work? It depends. Every year our best disease folks try to figure out which pirates are gonna pillage and plunder in the coming season. Over the last few years they've done a pretty good job at guessing right, but the Centers for Disease Control will be the first to admit that, frankly, in some years, the flu shot isn't worth diddly-squat.

The shot has been up to 70 percent effective; meaning of ten immunized folks exposed to flu, seven didn't get it at all, while three had some bad luck. Most years' effectiveness has been between 50 and 70 percent.

If your kiddo does have some bad luck and gets the flu anyway, having a flu shot will actually reduce the length and severity of the illness by giving the immune system a head start. Yeah, maybe it flunked out of flu school, but it remembered a thing or two, and that's better than starting with nothing. And reducing the length and severity of the flu also reduces the risk of scary complications like pneumonia and death.

The flu shot does have one overhyped side effect, used by some folks as an excuse not to get a shot for their kids: Guillain-Barré Syndrome, a rare muscle weakness and paralysis disorder, which is generally temporary. One in 100,000 people getting a flu shot are at risk, mostly older adults. That means for your kiddo, the flu risk hugely outweighs the Guillain-Barré risk.

continued on next page

UNDERSTANDING FLU, THE FLU SHOT, AND THE PIRATES OF THE CARIBBEAN con't

But I want you to get a flu shot, too. And your spouse. And your parents. And your in-laws. And your little type 1's sibs. Teamwork protects our most vulnerable.

And one last thought. Get the damn shots, but don't live in fear of the pirates. After all, it's kids first, diabetes (and flu) second.

Diabetes author, educator, and advocate William "Lee" Dubois, BS, AAS, CPT, is the Diabetes Coordinator for Pecos Valley Medical Center. He's has adult-onset type 1 diabetes and is the award-winning author of four books about diabetes.

CHAPTER TEN

All in the Family

A diagnosis of diabetes impacts the entire family—from parents trying to share added responsibilities, to siblings demanding more attention, and grandparents learning how to manage a whole new level of caregiving. Diabetes changes a family's life to the core. It can bring a family closer together or pull it apart. It takes a good deal of communication, understanding, and sometimes a little outside help, to maintain healthy family dynamics.

Captain of the Ship

As you've gathered, there is a tremendous amount of information and an equally large amount of stuff to juggle when a member of the family has diabetes. I think in most families, one parent, usually the one with the most flexible schedule, becomes the primary caregiver of the child with diabetes. It's not that the other parent is uninterested, but having one parent taking the wheel can oftentimes make the ship sail more smoothly. Frequently, the captain is the mother, but in some families, like that of Scott Benner who writes the blog Arden's Day (www.ardensday.com), the father can also take on this role.

The parent who takes the lead role becomes the go-to person. She (or he!) is the one the certified diabetes educator (CDE) from the endocrinologist's office calls to discuss recent blood sugar logs. That parent is the one the school calls first when the child has low or high blood sugar, or when unexpected giant birthday cupcakes suddenly appear at snack time. He or she is the one who can more often than not volunteer for school field trips when the nurse can't go. This designated person acts as the point of contact between the family and the medical team or endocrinologist.

Let's face it: family life is busy no matter how many kids you have, whether both parents work outside the home or one stays home, and with or without the added pressure of diabetes. Letting one parent take charge can streamline the long to-do list that comes with managing diabetes, like filling prescriptions as supplies dwindle, knowing and using the lingo that insurance companies understand, making appointments, and keeping up with ever-changing insulin-to-carb ratios and correction factors.

In our family, I have taken on the role of captain of the *S.S. Diabetes*. At times, I do feel overwhelmed because my head is swimming with blood sugar numbers, appointment dates, school lunch menus, and the latest research on treatments and technologies that are coming down the pike. Some families can find a good balance doling out responsibilities between the two parents. Find whatever works best for you, but no matter how the responsibilities are split, it's very important that both of you be on the same page regarding care and communicate often.

Sharing Responsibilities

Just because one of you is captain of the ship doesn't mean that you don't also need a first mate. You may have taken on the organizational role, but your partner has a job to do, too. Sometimes as one parent becomes the "expert" in diabetes care, the other finds it easier to step back and let the expert take over. To prevent this from happening, you need to find ways to keep your spouse involved.

Randy may not load the dishwasher as efficiently as I do, but I am happy that he's the one that does the dishes every day. Similarly, your spouse may not do all of the diabetes-related tasks exactly the way you would do them, but he or she needs to feel confident about being able, in fact, to do them. It's sometimes difficult for me not to step in and take over when Randy is changing Quinn's insulin pump site, but he needs to feel confident in her care, and more importantly, he needs to know that I'm confident he can take care of her. Your child also needs to feel safe and cared for by both of you.

After all, I am not with my daughter every minute of every day. In fact, Randy takes the kids camping and is primary caretaker when I travel. He has had his fair share of birthday party duty. I joke that he is a "stage dad" because he takes Quinn to a lot of her dance classes and skating lessons, and has volunteered at every recital so someone can stay with her backstage. He has even taken her to an endocrinology appointment without me when I couldn't go. (I may or may not have suggested he Skype me during the appointment so I could hear answers to the questions I wrote out. Needless to say, I didn't receive a call from him until after the appointment was over.)

If you would like to share responsibility with your spouse or distribute some of the tasks, think about areas that you could delegate. Share information about any variations in your child's

TWICE THE HOPE

Tim and Heather Brand

Having two children with type 1 diabetes is something we never thought we would be capable of handling. After the diagnosis of our middle child, Lovebug, in April of 2009, we knew the chance of having a second child diagnosed was increased. We just didn't believe it would become a reality. Then, in April of 2011, our greatest fear was confirmed—our youngest daughter, Princess, was also diagnosed.

Emotionally, it hit us HARD. Our emotions ran the gamut that day—we were shocked, sad, dumbfounded, and angry. It's hard to put into words what we were feeling (actually, what we are still feeling). And so we have begun our journey caring for two children with type 1 diabetes.

The hardest part of having Princess diagnosed with type 1 was knowing all the difficulties she would encounter on a daily basis. We already had two years of experience dealing with this medical condition, so her day-to-day care came far too easily to us. Even now there are days when our hearts and minds just want to dwell on the diagnosis. We relive that day and shed a lot of tears. Some days we feel like sulking, but we know we must keep pushing forward. Though it's difficult, we have tried our best to keep up with normal life. After all, we have to be the pancreas for two beautiful children.

People tell us they don't know how we do it. The reality is, like many challenging situations, you just do it. It's almost like flying on autopilot. You do whatever you have to do for your kids. Keeping our normal routine helped, so by the time the shock of the second diagnosis wore off, we realized we were already functioning.

Our friends, family, faith, and support network in the diabetes community helped carry us through those first few months. Other families, who had also gone through a second diagnosis, gave us great support. Soon, a daily routine developed, and diabetes became a part of life instead of an overwhelming task.

This has also been an adjustment for our oldest daughter, Peanut, who has a healthy pancreas. After her second sister was diagnosed, we knew she would be fearful of also being diagnosed. We did what we could to calm her anxiety. Tim bought her a bear dressed in a doctor's outfit to serve the same emotional role as Rufus (the Bear with Diabetes) does for our d-kids. Since Lovebug and Princess get a little more attention because of the diabetes, we try our best to spend time with just Peanut. We also lend a listening and sympathetic ear to her fears and thoughts about diabetes.

Through it all, our girls have been a great support to each other. Lovebug really encourages her youngest sister emotionally. She was the reason Princess wanted a pump so quickly after her diagnosis. Princess kept telling us from day one that she didn't want shots; she wanted a pump like her sister. We also try to find humor in the little things. Princess once told a friend of ours that she had "purple diabetes" because she was issued a purple pump! Despite their medical condition, they still act like normal sisters—squabbling, playing, and competing for attention. A connection has formed between them that we will never understand. We won't ever really know what it feels like to have high or low blood sugar, but they do. If there is any comfort in all of this, it's knowing they have each other for support and encouragement.

The second diagnosis has given us an even greater desire to be advocates for children with diabetes. We have become very passionate about advocacy and believe both parents, especially husbands, need to be more involved in daily care when there is a second diagnosis. We also feel compelled to reach out to families with newly diagnosed children to offer advice and understanding. Meeting other families who have children with type 1 was very comforting to us after our first diagnosis. We recognize that sometimes others simply need to see that another family with diabetes is functioning. It gives us hope. We enjoy sharing our experiences, and realize that sometimes words of encouragement and just knowing someone is there is what matters most.

Tim and Heather have three daughters, two of whom have type 1 diabetes. Their girls were diagnosed at ages 3 and 3 1/2. Tim and Heather both share the family's experiences on their blogs. Read Tim's perspective as a d-dad at his blog Bleeding Finger (www.bleedingfinger.com) and Heather's perspective as a d-mom at Sweet 2 the Soul (sweet2thesoul.blogspot.com).

care. When changes are made in your child's snack routine or how much insulin she or he receives, make sure to communicate these changes to your spouse. Keep current insulin-to-carb ratios and correction factors posted on the bulletin board so your spouse can easily double check.

And remember, you can't bear the entire burden of your child's diabetes care on your shoulders alone. You need the support of your spouse or other family members, and they will certainly rise to the occasion and do what is needed to help your child's diabetes management be successful. Sometimes it's just a matter of asking.

Couple Time

Date night? What's that?

It's difficult enough to find a babysitter and have "couple time" when you have children who don't have a medical condition, but parents of children with diabetes often have a hard time letting someone else be the caretaker, even if it's only for a few hours so the two of you can have dinner and see a movie. As in any marriage, it's important to have some one-on-one time when you can focus on each other, share a bottle of wine, and decompress. Of course, you'll probably be checking your phone the entire time to see if the babysitter called, but it's good to give it a try.

We are fortunate that my parents can act as our babysitters on the occasions that we have a night on the town. My mom is familiar with Quinn's care; after all, she did watch her every day until she went to kindergarten. She still calls with questions since she's not entrenched in the day-to-day care anymore. Last New Year's Eve both kids had a sleepover at their grandparents'. Randy and I caught a matinee, had dinner at a wine bar, and were back home by 8:45 PM! That's how you can tell you are getting older!

If you are looking for a babysitter, put the feelers out to other families of children with diabetes you know; maybe they have found a good one already. Siblings of d-kids and teens and college students with

> ! If you are nervous about leaving your child with a new babysitter, do a dry run with the babysitter by staying at home and being productive elsewhere in the house or run errands nearby so you can come home if really necessary.

diabetes will be quick to learn how you do things for your own child. If your child attends diabetes camp in the summer, take note if any of the counselors live in your area. You can also post job announcements on the website of the local college and may even find a nursing student. Another idea is to trade babysitting with another family who has a child with diabetes.

Don't Forget the Siblings

When Quinn was diagnosed, her brother Rowan was just shy of his first birthday. He will never remember her before she had diabetes. He is used to the daily care she receives, including all the blood sugar checks and insulin pump changes. He knows about all the work that goes into putting a meal on the table and knowing how much insulin to give her for it. For him, it's part of our family life.

But that's not to say that it doesn't affect him. Because diabetes management takes so much of your time and focus, it's easy for the non-diabetic child to feel left out or deprived of your time. What you don't want is for the other child to feel neglected and to start acting out at home or school as a way to get your attention.

You may be able to find some ways to involve the other child in the daily diabetes routine, though you don't want it to become a burden or something to worry about. Quinn never had a bedtime snack before she was diagnosed, and we probably wouldn't have offered it to Rowan. But he likes to sit at the table with her and have a bedtime snack, as well. Although we have a stash of juice boxes, Smarties, and glucose tablets that are for treating blood sugar only, he sometimes asks for a juice box, a roll of Smarties, or even a glucose tablet when Quinn gets one. Sometimes I indulge him.

If you have an incentive chart for your child with diabetes, say as a reward for getting injections or changing her insulin pump site,

TRIALNET NATURAL HISTORY STUDY

One question that comes up often with siblings is "Does type 1 diabetes run in families?" The answer is no. Families that have a member with type 1 diabetes do have a higher chance of another family member being diagnosed with it, but the chance is still so low that it is not expected. There is only about a 2 to 5 percent risk of a sibling also having type 1. For families who want to know, there are studies that can detect whether siblings, and other family members, carry the antibodies for possible development. The study, called TrialNet (www.diabetestrialnet.org) looks for three different antibodies.

According to their website, "Type 1 Diabetes TrialNet is an international network of researchers who are exploring ways to prevent, delay, and reverse the progression of type 1 diabetes." The group is conducting two types of clinical studies in 18 centers in the United States and throughout the world, in addition to over 150 participating medical offices. The Pathway to Prevention Study "provide(s) information about risk factors associated with developing type 1 diabetes," while the Diabetes Intervention Studies "test either treatments to delay or prevent the onset of type 1 diabetes, or test treatments to preserve remaining insulin secretion in people recently diagnosed with type 1 diabetes."

Screening is a simple blood draw and is performed on relatives between 1 and 45 years of age who have a sibling, child, or parent with type 1 diabetes, think of something your other child could do to earn stickers or other incentives. This praise will make him feel like he's accomplishing something, too.

The non-diabetic sibling might feel lost in the commotion, so it's a good idea to spend some one-on-one time with him or her. Maybe take turns taking non-diabetic siblings to a movie, the park, or the local children's museum to provide some alone time—time where there is absolutely no diabetes care taking your attention. Make them your focus for those few hours.

and relatives between 1 and 20 years of age who have a cousin, aunt, uncle, niece, nephew, half sibling or grandparent with type 1 diabetes. With the blood draw, clinicians are looking for diabetes-related autoantibodies.

Our family was at a diabetes event where TrialNet was conducting blood draws. My husband and I opted to each get tested, though we chose not to test our four-year-old for a couple of reasons. First, having the diabetes-related autoantibody doesn't guarantee that a person will develop diabetes in his or her lifetime, and we didn't want to spend our lives worrying and looking for signs and symptoms. Some families want siblings to be tested to either give them reassurance that the antibody isn't present or to help prepare them for the possibility. Second, we were at an amusement park and didn't want to ruin our son's day.

A month later my husband and I both received letters stating that we do not have the antibody. We were both happy to contribute to the clinical trial, and will let our son choose to participate when he is old enough to decide for himself.

I personally feel this study is important because the other aspect, the Diabetes Intervention Studies, is investigating ways to delay or prevent the onset of type 1 diabetes in those at risk and to preserve insulin production in newly diagnosed children.

Rowan is still too young to understand a lot of the medical aspects of diabetes and why his sister has it, but he has mentioned several times that he wishes he had diabetes like Quinn. While I wanted to say "No, no you don't," I also don't want either child to feel like it's something to be jealous of or that Quinn is somehow deficient. I think the best thing I can do is talk with him about his feelings and try to understand where he is coming from. I will say that one of the bedtime stories we have read over and over is *Mickey Mouse Clubhouse: Coco and Goofy's Goofy Day* in which their friend Coco, who has type 1 diabetes, comes to his birthday party. Rowan always talks about the bad choices that Goofy makes at the party. Interestingly, he always wants me to read the Q&A at the end of the book, which addresses why Coco needs to check her blood sugar and what she carries in her supply bag. I think reading this story repeatedly helps him come to terms with it in an age-appropriate way. Or maybe he just really likes Mickey Mouse books.

My son isn't old enough yet to worry about his sister's diabetes. But I am sure there will come a time when he will begin to ask if he, too, may develop diabetes or he may become fearful that his sister could become sick or even die. When he begins to have questions or fears, we will talk with him in age-appropriate terms to assure him that he doesn't need to worry because as his mom and dad, we will always do our best to take care of the both of them and help them to be as healthy as they can be.

Extended Family

If it takes a village to raise a typical child, then d-parents really need help! When your child is first diagnosed, many family members might want to lend you a hand, but they may not know how.

If you need an extra pair of hands, take advantage of offers. Family members can run errands for you, go shopping, babysit while you take a much-needed nap, or even stock your freezer with a few meals ... though you'll probably be guessing at the carb counts and serving sizes. As time passes, friends and family may not think you need help, because on the surface you look like you have everything under control. However, diabetes care is a marathon, not a sprint. You'll have an entire lifetime of dealing with diabetes and support from family and friends can help ease your load.

When Quinn was diagnosed, my mom was thrust into the role of providing care for her because she cared for the children while I worked. The children's hospital suggested that she come in for training, too. Ask your endocrinologist if the office offers training or classes for grandparents or aunts and uncles who not only want to learn about the medical condition, but could also benefit from the confidence that education will give them.

Invite extended family to local support group meetings and encourage them to get involved in your fundraising and advocacy work, such as annual diabetes walks. It will make them feel that they are making a contribution. Conferences such as the *Children With Diabetes—Friends For Life*, held annually in July in Orlando, Florida, even have a grandparents track where they can learn about topics specific to the role they might play in your child's care. Plus, they will meet other grandparents with whom they can share their feelings and look to for support.

ADVENTURES IN BABYSITTING

Allison Blass

The idea of spending a night alone with your spouse after your child is diagnosed with diabetes might seem like a foreign concept. How could you leave your child alone with someone who doesn't understand the intricacies of blood sugar readings, carb counts, and insulin doses? When I started baby-sitting children with diabetes in high school, I had many parents tell me what a "godsend" I was and that I was a "lifesaver" for babysitting their child. I quickly learned that an educated, experienced babysitter (I was diagnosed with type 1 at age eight) was in high demand, and I occasionally traveled 30 minutes to some of my clients! Even though I'm in my mid-twenties and married (no children just yet!), I still occasionally babysit for families with children with diabetes because I have seen firsthand what a struggle it is for parents.

When I was growing up, my parents did not have a babysitter with diabetes. Like most folks, we had a teenager from our neighborhood watch my brother and me. She had no experience with diabetes, but she was willing to learn, so my parents and I taught her what I needed to do to manage my diabetes. Now, for some of you this will be easier than others. Managing diabetes in a toddler is much different than managing diabetes in a fifth grader. If you're lucky enough to have someone in your immediate circle with diabetes, hang on to that person! If you don't, I have some tips for finding a trusted babysitter to help take care of your child. It may seem impossible, but it isn't. Like all things in diabetes, it just takes a little extra work. Here are some tips:

- I have been babysitting children with diabetes for 10 years. One of my biggest strengths? I have had diabetes for almost 20 years. My first tip is to look for a babysitter who already has knowledge about diabetes. There are several places you can look:
  - Ask your local chapter of JDRF or ADA if they have any teen volunteers in your area.
  - Talk to your CDE or endocrinologist to find out if there are patients interested in babysitting.
  - If there is a local diabetes camp, talk to the camp director about counselors or counselors-in-training who may live nearby.

- Inquire with a local nursing school if there are any students interested in babysitting a child with special needs.
- Safesittings.com specializes in diabetes, and Childrenwithdiabetes.com's Family Support Network can help connect families with a babysitter. I have had luck finding clients using Safesittings. You can either post an ad about your family, or you can search for a babysitter in your area.

- If you can't find a babysitter who has diabetes or experience with diabetes, you can use traditional methods like word-of-mouth, fliers at schools, or online services like Sittercity to find a babysitter who is willing to learn. Another option is to ask a family member or close friend.
- Once you find someone you're comfortable with, I recommend meeting with the sitter before you even schedule a night on the town. Invite him or her over to meet you and your family. (I recommend at least some compensation for their time.) While the sitter is there:
  - Explain your child's typical evening/weekend routine.
  - Show them where the diabetes supplies, juice, and emergency supplies are located.
  - Demonstrate how a glucose meter, insulin pen, or insulin pump works.
  - Depending on your babysitter, discuss what kind of emergency plan you will have; decide whether you will come home if an insulin pump site falls off or if there is more than one high blood sugar reading in a row.
  - Write up simple instructions with the basic information that a babysitter would need to know for the time frame you'll be gone.
  - Even though I have lived with diabetes for more than half my life and have watched dozens of children with diabetes, I still visit a family prior to my first time babysitting for them. Parents are often a little too frazzled getting ready for their night out and saying

continued on next page

ADVENTURES IN BABYSITTING con't

good-bye to their child to give me all the information I need. Every child is different, and all children have their own preferred ways of treating a low. There may also be a meter or insulin pump that I'm not as familiar with.

- If you're very concerned about leaving your child alone with someone new, have your babysitter come over for some supervised time with your child (paid, of course). Not only does this help the child get used to the babysitter, but it also gives the babysitter time to manage your child's diabetes with you in the other room if there is a question or concern.

- Remember, the idea of a night out is to relax and spend some quality time with your significant other. Keep in contact via text or a quick phone call, but try to limit the frequency and length. This will become easier to do the more familiar your babysitter becomes with diabetes and your child. When I'm getting to know a family, I try to limit my conversations with parents to just the blood sugar reading, or if I have a question. After a while, I get to know the child's diabetes and the parents learn to trust me. Trust takes time to develop, and it develops through communication.

Allison Blass was diagnosed with type 1 diabetes 18 years ago at age 8. In addition to her special babysitting talents, Allison is an assistant editor at DiabetesMine.com.

CHAPTER ELEVEN

Your Support System

You cannot do this alone. Parenting a child with type 1 diabetes can be a lonely road, but you don't have to travel it by yourself. There are thousands of people out there making the same journey. Besides the support of your family and your medical team, there are numerous resources available. While a great deal of focus is put on technological advances, don't underestimate the importance of the human connection. Nothing is as powerful as sharing firsthand experiences and finding a kindred spirit who "gets it."

A Positive Outlook

Dealing with diabetes day in and day out can really take a toll on a parent. We are exhausted from disrupted sleep schedules, zombie our way through work days, and somehow juggle the activities and demands of family life. At times, it can be overwhelming, but having a strong support system can help you avoid burnout and save your sanity. Remember, you need to be strong and healthy so you can care for your child. Doctors can give great medical advice, but nobody knows how to deal with diabetes better than the people who live with it every day.

Now, I'm not saying that life with diabetes is all rainbows and unicorns, but I do believe in the power of a positive outlook. I have never taken the attitude "woe is me." I don't wallow in my misery, and I certainly don't want my child to look at the negative side of things all the time.

I think the key is to take control, but I don't mean it in the way you normally hear the word control associated with diabetes (i.e., keeping blood sugar in a tight range). For me, taking control means coming to terms with your child's diagnosis and accepting it. It means getting organized and streamlining your systems so that management isn't so taxing; automating as much as you can as I described in the chapters about organizing supplies; figuring out carb counts for foods and recipes and writing it down so you don't have to figure it out again; and making charts with insulin to carb ratios and correction factors to reduce your math. Taking control means getting on with life and not letting diabetes hold you or your child back.

I don't know how many times a well-meaning person has asked me if Quinn's diabetes is "under control." What does that even mean? Anyone who has firsthand experience with diabetes knows you can't control it. While there is a ton of diabetes math we must do each day, the reality is that with diabetes, one plus one does not always equal two. I think that's one of the hardest things for parents of newly diagnosed children to understand. You can do the same exact thing three days in a row, and on one of those days you may have a completely different outcome. Giving the same amount of insulin for the identical meal or blood sugar may have a different result each time, because there are so many other factors that affect how the body uses insulin and food, such as exercise, activity, illness, growth, stress, and more.

Here are some of my best pieces of advice for parents of children with diabetes:

- You can't control diabetes 100 percent of the time, but you should strive to do the best you can.
- Make the best decisions you can with the knowledge you have at the time.
- Of course, hindsight is 20/20, but you can't beat yourself up for not knowing everything about diabetes management from day one.
- Forgive yourself for the few times you get it wrong. Look at how many times you get it right!
- Learn by experience. If you find that a certain food or activity affects your child in a certain way, make a note of it and try it differently the next time. Better yet, ask your CDE or endocrinologist for suggestions.
- Fear is not a good motivator. Looking at potential negative outcomes will not make you or your child want to try your best.
- Let that guilt go. I know that's easier said than done. You did nothing to cause this, and you couldn't have prevented it.
- Know when it's worth educating others and when you should ignore them. Try not to get too upset by ignorance.
- Take things one blood sugar at a time. Sometimes it's all we have in us to do.
- Tomorrow is a fresh start with a clean slate.

I think this quote sums up my philosophy when it comes to managing diabetes without guilt: "*Finish each day and be done with it. You have done what you could. Some blunders and absurdities have crept in; forget them as soon as you can. Tomor-row is a new day. You shall begin it serenely and with too high a spirit to be encumbered with your old nonsense."* —Emerson

The Stages of Grief

I'll admit that when Quinn was diagnosed, I instantly went into what I call "mom mode" as my way of coping and getting done what needed to be done in those first few weeks and months. At her first follow-up visit, three months after diagnosis, a psychologist came into the room and asked Quinn a few questions. She asked me how I was doing, and with a shaky voice I replied, "Fine." I knew that if I said anything more I would likely break down crying, something I didn't want to do in front of Quinn.

From Dr. Elisabeth Kübler-Ross's book *On Death and Dying* that I read for a college psychology class, I remember the stages of grief—denial, anger, bargaining, depression, and acceptance. Though a diagnosis of diabetes in your child is not a diagnosis of death, I think it's important that we allow ourselves to go through these stages of grief in order to accept and heal. If you think about it, we do need to mourn a loss. Our children's lives and our family life will never be the same. The lives we imagined for them will not be as easy as we would like them to be. They will have times of emotional and financial struggle because of diabetes. They will lose some of their childhood innocence and ability to be carefree.

You may not need to go through all the stages, and you may not go through them in the same order. Though I don't think I was ever in denial, I have met many parents who are in those first few weeks. I bet every one of us has tried to make a bargain, saying we would take it away from our children and put it on ourselves in a heartbeat. I know I go through waves of minor depression when I cry easily out of frustration with diabetes or from extreme fatigue. But, I believe I have come to terms with diabetes and have found acceptance.

So, when I say that days go by without thinking about diabetes, it's both true and false. It's a part of every minute of our lives. It's ingrained in our routine. We constantly pack the heavy bag before leaving the house and dutifully lug it with us. We test her blood sugar and give her insulin. We count carbs. We weigh and measure food. We read labels. We pack snacks. We fill prescriptions and calculate insulin dosages. We awake at 2:00 in the morning to check her finger while she sleeps to make sure she isn't going low. It has become so habitual, that it's just a part of life now. And yet, there are still moments when it hits me like a ton of bricks. Overall, I have come to terms with it, have accepted it for what it is, and can make the best of our lives with diabetes. I hope you are in that place, too, or are on a path to get there.

The Dreaded A1c (a.k.a. the Report Card)

I have probably said a dozen times in this book that you need to do the best you can, given the knowledge you have at the time. I have also said that sometimes you need to take diabetes one blood sugar at a time. There is a tremendous amount of guilt that comes along with caring for a child with diabetes, and you find yourself questioning whether you are really doing the best you can for your child.

The fact remains: we are not pancreases. Even with education, training, and fancy charts to dictate every action and reaction when it comes to diabetes care, we just can't do the job of a perfectly functioning pancreas. When a number pops up on a glucose meter or your endocrinologist tells you what your child's A1c is, you cannot take that as an assessment of your parenting skills. They are just numbers. These numbers are tools that we should use to make decisions. You take that number and react appropriately. But don't take it personally, no matter how difficult it is.

So that guess you made as to the number of carbs you gave your child was way off, and now she's in the 300s. Bolus and move on. You did the best you could at the time. Make a mental note, or leave an actual note on your bulletin board or log book, for the next time she eats that same meal that you need to count it as more carbs.

So that A1c was a full point higher than you thought. Talk with your endocrinologist and develop a game plan. Review your logbook with him or her to identify trends. Maybe you need to adjust basal rates or long-acting insulin dosages, maybe mealtime ratios need changing. But sometimes that A1c is completely out of your control because of growth spurts, or illness, or who the heck knows what! I know you want to cry all the way home because you think you have failed your child, but really, you haven't. Don't judge your parenting skills by the A1c. It's not a grade.

> Take on diabetes one meal and one blood sugar at a time.

Finding a Therapist

Maintaining a happy, healthy marriage and a busy family can be difficult enough on its own. When you add in the stressors that diabetes brings—physical and mental exhaustion, financial costs of care including insurance premiums, supplies, and prescriptions, and all the extra work involved just to get a meal on the table—of course tensions can rise on the home front. If you, your child, or your family is struggling, it's okay to take the next step and find a therapist.

We all know that arguments usually aren't about the stupid thing being argued about. You might feel resentment toward a spouse who you don't feel is carrying his or her weight. You may feel paralyzed by grief or completely overwhelmed by the daily diabetes tasks that are stacked up on top of all the other things that must get done each day. A therapist can help you work through your feelings and come to terms with the diabetes diagnosis, give you coping skills to help you get through the day, and open up communication between you and your spouse, so the two of you can more effectively manage your relationship and your family. If you need help coping, don't be afraid to ask. Your medical team may be able to recommend a qualified therapist.

Finding Support

There are many places to look for support. Whether you go the traditional route and find people in your own community or reach out to others online, it's important you find others who "get it." While only a small percentage of the population has type 1 diabetes, you might be surprised at how many parents of children and adults with type 1 diabetes you can find if you just put your feelers out there.

In Person

It can be a very powerful and meaningful experience to meet

with other parents who know what you're going through, whether you need answers to questions, or simply want to share your concerns with someone who understands. Some hospitals that have pediatric endocrinology departments offer regular support groups for parents and families. If the hospital or endocrinology practice you are using doesn't have one, ask them if they can refer you to a local support group. In addition, you can find support groups through local chapters of organizations such as the ADA or JDRF. They may also be able to assign you a mentor or put you in touch with other local families.

You can also start your own informal support system. I know a group of moms who try to get together once a month for dinner and a glass of wine. They chat for hours, mostly sharing their experiences dealing with diabetes, including school, sports, and the pumps and CGMs they are using. It's great to be able to ask questions and learn how others do things. Sometimes they have better answers than the "experts" because they are in the trenches.

Online

The nice thing about the Internet is that it's there every minute of the day. I can log onto Facebook or Twitter at 2:00 AM, and there is another mom or dad or adult T1 awake and dealing with diabetes with whom I can commiserate. The number of diabetes-related blogs is growing exponentially, and you are sure to find a few that suit your tastes. The first time you read a blog and realize there is someone else out there who "gets it" is like an epiphany.

When you're ready, you might consider starting your own blog. I find it to be quite cathartic to write about my feelings and experiences and get it all out. It's also an easy way to develop friendships with other parents when you begin commenting on each other's blogs.

In addition to blogs, there are several online communities where you can connect with others, add people as friends or contacts to interact more deeply, and join groups with similar interests, such as insulin pump users, or people living in a certain region or state. These online communities also have forums that allow you to ask questions and get answers or have a discussion on a topic. If you are looking for an online community, here are some places to start:

- TuDiabetes, www.tudiabetes.org/
- Children With Diabetes, www.childrenwithdiabetes.com/
- Juvenation (JDRF), www.juvenation.org

My one caveat, which should really go without saying, is to remember that just because you're on a computer doesn't mean you should forget your values or your manners. Unfortunately, there are some people who are negative forces. As with dealings in person, it's best to surround yourself with people online who lift you up, rather than bring you down. There are many of us out there!

SOMETIMES GETTING IT WRONG

Stacey Simms

My son was diagnosed at 23 months, a little more than five years ago. While we've been dealing with diabetes for a while, we still never know when it's going to throw a curve ball our way, or when we'll

continued on next page

SOMETIMES GETTING IT WRONG con't

accidently drop the ball. Managing diabetes is a 24/7 undertaking.

It helps to have incredible technology like my son's insulin pump, but it doesn't make the process automatic.

Last summer offers a good example. On a record-breaking 101-degree day I took my son and daughter out to lunch and then let them run around in a nearby splash fountain. We were prepared—bathing suits on, insulin pump off. It's very easy to remove; Benny disconnected, handed it over, and ran to play. The kids had a great time; they cooled off and we all spent the afternoon inside at home, trying to beat the heat.

Seemed like another typical summer day until the mid-afternoon blood sugar check. It was a shocker: 500 mg/dL. Just what did he eat at lunch? Did I miss something? I used our new Animas Ping to give Benny a big bolus of insulin. The Ping has a cool remote control we'd received just six weeks earlier. We loved it right away; no more touching the pump, it's all wireless. We heard the pump whirring away, delivering. All better, right?

Wrong. An hour later Benny said he didn't feel well. At this check we got the dreaded HIGH GLUCOSE reading. We don't see that very often, but when we do, I always feel like the meter is yelling at us. (We know there's a problem—you don't have to shout.)

That off-the-charts reading required immediate action. I asked Benny if he felt the bolus go in. Sometimes he doesn't, but he said he had, both times. Then I told him we needed to take a look at the connection, maybe it wasn't fully clicked in? I'll say—it wasn't there at all. No pump! I had forgotten to click it back on after the fountain run four hours earlier.

You've got to be kidding me. I found the pump inside my purse, which had apparently received all that insulin. When we thought about it, I realized that Benny had been standing right next to my purse, which explains why we'd heard the pump working. I still don't know what he thought he felt—a phantom bolus?

Not realizing Benny might not be wearing his pump could be one slight drawback to using a remote control. I resolved to just pay more attention; after all, this isn't something I could remember ever happening to us in five years of diabetes management.

Besides, Benny loves the remote. It's easier for him or anyone to administer insulin. He wears his pump on his hip, and he's old enough now that he really doesn't want anyone reaching over and fussing with his waistband! So even though I had used it to bolus my purse, we didn't spend much time worrying whether the Ping remote was a keeper. Of course we'd keep using it.

Then I broke it. Yes, I did. Just a few minutes after we'd reunited Benny and his pump, the remote just slipped out of my hands and landed on our wood floor. Crack. Aaargh!

Not my day. Animas agreed to send a replacement Ping, but I felt horrible. I felt guilty for messing up Benny's day, and for breaking his new meter. Just awful.

I also felt alone. I took my frustration to Twitter; the first time I'd ever shared something "bad" about our experience with diabetes. I explained what had happened and how awful I was feeling. Right away, I got some great responses.

How cool is that? Within minutes, I felt better. Still mad and frustrated, but no longer alone. I was grateful for those responses and so very glad I reached out.

Later that evening, Benny's blood sugar was back to normal and he was feeling good. It only took two days for the new meter to arrive in the mail. Back to the business of managing diabetes in its messy, confusing, gotta-be-alert-around-the-clock sort of way. That doesn't change. I'm not sure it ever will.

What did change for me that day is the knowledge that we never have to face diabetes alone; someone who "gets it" is always just a click away. The next time you feel like you're in this by yourself, I urge you to reach out. Connect. Just keep a firm grip on your meter while you do so!

Stacey Simms is the host of Charlotte's Morning News on NewsTalk 1110 WBT radio and the author of I Can't Cook, But I Know Someone Who Can (all profits donated to JDRF). Her son was diagnosed with type 1 diabetes in 2006 at 23 months. Stacey is on the Board of the Charlotte chapter of JDRF and she blogs about diabetes at www.staceysimms.com.

CHAPTER TWELVE

Comfort for Kids

Just as you need help to cope, support is even more important for your child with diabetes. In addition to the added responsibilities and constant planning, your child may feel like the only child in the world with this medical condition. At times, children may think that no one else gets it, or that diabetes will keep them from reaching for the stars. But your child doesn't have to feel alone in this.

Why Your Child Needs Support

As we parents come to terms with the diabetes diagnosis, it's important that our kids be allowed to grieve and find acceptance, too. Not quite a year after her diagnosis, we left a birthday party, and as we drove past a familiar building Quinn said, "Remember when daddy worked in that building and he took me on a tour? I wasn't diabetic when he worked there." The conversation went on and culminated with the following:

Quinn: Why do I have diabetes?

Me: Some kids have diabetes and some don't. Unfortunately, we don't have a choice.

Quinn: But we do have a choice, and I choose not to be diabetic.

Me: I'm sorry, but it's not that simple and not our choice to make.

What do you say to a four-year-old saddled with a condition many adults have difficulty handling? That was the first time she asked me why she had diabetes, but not the last. As I continued driving, tears came to my eyes because there was really nothing I could say or do to take it away from her. I cried quietly most of the way to our destination, glad that she was seated behind me out of view, putting on the happiest voice I could as our banter continued on a different subject. That's what it's like for her. She takes it all in stride. After a bad moment, she gets on with her life.

Sometimes it feels like she has had diabetes forever. Other times, I remember the pre-diagnosis freedom, and it seems like only yesterday that we were carefree. But we have to live our lives. We have to be constantly prepared for the worst, but we have to live.

I am sure your child has asked the same question about why he or she has diabetes. It's a difficult question for parents to answer because there really is nothing we could have done to keep our child from getting diabetes. And, of course, we would take it away if we could.

While we can't take it away, there are things we can do to help our children cope and adjust. As I mentioned in the last chapter, if your child is struggling you may need to look into professional help. Endocrinology practices often have a psychologist on staff that can help children make the adjustment and deal with their feelings. You might be able to work a short counseling session into your regularly scheduled visit. Alternatively, you can seek out separate counseling.

Whether your child talks to a professional, to friends who also

RUFUS THE BEAR WITH DIABETES

When our daughter was diagnosed, we were told by the nurses to contact the JDRF for a teddy bear. As we settled in back home, I eventually e-mailed our state's JDRF chapter to request our Bag of Hope. They mailed it with lightning speed, and I think we received it two days later.

And that was a good thing.

Quinn had been pretty compliant about finger checks and injections up until that point. But all of a sudden, about a month out post-diagnosis, she decided she just was not having it any more.

Injections were accompanied by screaming and tears from her and threats from me that she could do it the easy way or the hard way. I had to demand that she could sit still and make it quick, or I could hold her down, which would drag it out. However, there was no choice whether or not to get an injection.

This rebellion made for a difficult few days. I don't blame her. She was three and had every right to be fed up. But I didn't know what to do to get over this hump.

And then Rufus arrived, as if summoned by her d-fairy godmother.

We read the book about the little boy who was diagnosed with diabetes and his special bear. And then we practiced checking Rufus' finger and giving him an injection. And it worked!

No more struggles. No more tears. No more screaming. No more trying to get away from the needle that was coming toward her.

She still plays with Rufus, occasionally wanting to do his finger check or give him an injection. She doctors him up when he is feeling sick. She's repaired broken limbs and covered him in countless bandages. And when we were thinking about starting an insulin pump, she hooked Rufus up to a pump, too. Sometimes having a diabetes buddy can really help.

have diabetes, or to a teddy bear, it's important to be able to get his or her feelings out. Pent-up emotions can lead to depression. Children have a lifetime of dealing with diabetes ahead, and it's probably best to help them come to terms with it early on.

Don't be surprised if from time to time your child asks again why he or she got diabetes. As they grow and mature, children's understanding of diabetes and life in general will grow and mature. New situations, new friends, and new activities may bring up old feelings again. Be open to discussing their feelings and offer support, even if all you can say is, "I understand."

Forming a Community

I think one of the ways that kids can feel most comfortable about their diabetes is to meet other children with diabetes and form friendships. Nobody can understand their feelings better than another child who walks the same path as they do. I know Quinn always gets incredibly excited when she meets other kids, and even adults, with diabetes. It's almost like an exclusive club. And because I don't know what it's like to personally have diabetes, it's good for her to be around others who "get it" in the same way.

Where can your child meet other kids with diabetes? Invite other children with diabetes from school or church to join you for a playdate at a local park. Allow the kids some time to chat privately. They may talk about diabetes, or they may not. The grown-ups can share experiences while the kids play. Local support groups are a great place to meet other families and form friendships, too.

There are online resources available for kids of varying ages. Juvenation is a social network created by JDRF for people

DIABETES CAMPS

Kerri Morrone Sparling

Growing up, I was the only kid with diabetes that I knew. Diagnosed just before I started second grade, this strange world of insulin injections, glucose meters, and viewing juice as "medicine" was entirely new to my family and me ... and it was isolating. In that first year post-diagnosis, we spent a lot of time in hospitals and doctor's offices, learning the ropes of this new disease, but not a lot of time connecting with other families who were experiencing the same learning curve. We learned the basics, but had no idea how things looked in "real life." Where were all the other kids who were shooting up before breakfast, like I did every morning?

Even then, as a little kid, I needed a community. Diabetes is a very physiological disease with the lack of insulin production and the delicate dance of blood sugar management, but it's also a frightfully psychological disease. You need to be emotionally on your game in order to best manage this disease, and emotional health is crucial to good diabetes health. Almost immediately after diagnosis, I was searching for people who understood. My parents tried, but couldn't despite their very best efforts. Clara Barton Camp (CBC) in North Oxford, Massachusetts, provided that sense of community that I craved.

Almost everyone at Barton had type 1 diabetes: all the campers, almost every counselor, and the majority of the staff. If your pancreas made insulin, you were the odd-man-out. Waking up in the morning and pricking your finger was normal. Carrying a cellophane-wrapped package of crackers and some glucose tabs was normal. Taking an injection of insulin every few hours was normal. The counselors would break out the big plastic tubs filled with blood sugar meters, syringes, bottles of insulin, and assorted

208

hypoglycemia treatment methods, and we'd all sit on the bunks and test. Or shoot. Or eat something.

And it was completely *normal*.

There's so much power to knowing you aren't alone, and that you can truly do this. Clara Barton Camp, like most diabetes camps, has this way of making you feel like you're being hugged the entire time you're there. It sounds cheesy, but it's true. CBC is like a second home to so many girls with diabetes, and for some, it's the first place they've ever felt like everything was going to be okay.

Sending me to camp was the best thing my parents ever did for me as their child with diabetes. Clara Barton Camp was where I felt normal, where this whole diabetes thing was normal. Looking back, I'm so proud of my mother for making the decision to sign me up for diabetes camp. I was barely a year out from being diagnosed with diabetes, but she understood that eventually the disease would be mine to manage ... and mine to make peace with. She knew I needed this.

Away from my family and friends for twelve days, I was surrounded by girls with whom I laughed immediately, but learned to trust enough to cry with, too. They were my diabetes family, the community that I craved, and the support I needed to keep diabetes from defining me.

Clara Barton Camp was my solace; it truly is the most wonderful place in the world.

Kerri Sparling was diagnosed with type 1 diabetes when she was seven. In 2005, she started Six Until Me, a website that provides honest, anecdotal information and support for individuals with type 1 diabetes. She is a freelance writer, public speaker, and shares her experience on her blog (www.SixUntilMe.com).

ages 13 and older with type 1 diabetes. Within the site, there are many special interest groups that you and your child can join. JDRF staff and volunteers monitor the site, but with all things Internet, I suggest monitoring your own child's online activity and deciding what age is appropriate for online interaction.

One of the best ways for children to meet other d-kids is by going to diabetes camp. There are a variety of diabetes camps throughout the country, including family camps, day camps, and overnight camps. There are also a number of sports camps, like snowboarding and basketball, geared toward type 1 kids.

Quinn will be going to diabetes camp this year for the first time. She began counting down the days a full five months in advance, and she started packing her suitcase in February for the July camp! The previous summer we had an opportunity to visit the camp and eat lunch with the rest of the campers. The camp she will attend has 12 campers per cabin and eight staff members, including a physician, nurse, and dietitian ... in each cabin! I wish we had that level of medical care at home. When we left, I half joked that I was fully confident in the medical care she would receive, but was a little worried about the bunk beds.

We saw firsthand that campers are at ease with each other because they all have diabetes, and it's a perfectly natural activity to check blood sugar and get injections. In fact, many of the staff members also have diabetes. At drop-off, parents help set a couple of goals for the children for the week to make them more self-sufficient in their care. Some goals are checking their own blood sugar, counting carbs, figuring out boluses, giving themselves injections, and changing their own pump or CGM sites. Diabetes camp can empower them by giving them the tools and confidence to manage their diabetes. Quinn has said she wants to learn how to bolus using her pump while at camp this summer.

Of course camp isn't all about diabetes. There is crafting, sports, campfires (complete with s'mores), dancing, and lots of other activities. And I hear over and over again that deep friendships are formed that continue for years, if not a lifetime.

Celebrate Diabetes

That's right, I said we should celebrate. When the one-year anniversary of my child's diagnosis came, I didn't mark the occasion. After interacting with people I had met online, I realized that celebrating small victories can really help us get through this with a more positive attitude. Many people mark their d-anniversaries, also called diaversaries by some, by having cupcakes, which I am finding is a very popular dessert among people with diabetes. (Just remember to bolus for them!) Anniversaries of the diagnosis date don't have to be somber occasions; rather, I like to think that we are marking yet another year of living ... and living well, despite diabetes.

There are other milestones you can mark with your child. Perhaps you use a sticker chart as an incentive for them to take on a certain diabetes task? The reward doesn't have to be a large one, but filling that chart and saying "job well done" can go a long way.

I know I've said there are no bad blood sugar or good blood sugar numbers, but some people like to play a little game with their meters. Every time a "100" pops up on Quinn's meter we take a photo of her showing off that perfect number. Some parents give their child a dollar for every 100. Of course, that's an

DIABETES CHAMPIONS

Your child with diabetes can do anything they set their mind to. Here is just a sample of the positive role models that your child might relate and look up to. No matter what your child's interests or passions, you are sure to find a person with type 1 diabetes who is paving the way … if not, maybe your child will be the first!

Athletes

Nick Boyton	NHL hockey player
Sean Busby	Professional snowboarder
Bill Carlson	First diabetic ironman triathlete
Jay Cutler	Chicago Bears quarterback
Tony Cervati	Endurance mountain biker
Will Cross	Mountain climber
Chris Dudley	NBA basketball player
Scott Dunton	Professional surfer
Joe Eldridge	"Race Across America" cyclist
Gary Forbes	NBA basketball player
Missy Foy	Marathon runner
Kris Freeman	Olympic cross country skier
Sam Fuld	Professional baseball player
Gary Hall Jr.	Olympic swimmer
Jay Hewitt	Ironman triathlete
Chris Jarvis	Champion rower
Zippora Karz	New York City Ballet soloist
Kelli Kuehne	LPGA golfer
Mark Lowe	Professional baseball player
Michelle McGann	LPGA golfer
Adam Morrison	Professional baseball player
Brandon Morrow	Professional baseball player
Matt Neal	BMX racer
David Pember	Professional baseball player
Toby Petersen	NHL hockey player

Dan Reichert	Professional baseball player
Sébastien Sasseville	Climbed Mount Everest, ironman triathlete
Cliff Scherb	Ironman triathlete
Ryan Shafer	Professional bowler
Phil Southerland	Professional cyclist, founder of Team Type 1
Scott Verplank	PGA golfer
Ginger Vieira	15-time record-setting powerlifter

Pop Culture

Crystal Bowersox	Singer and "American Idol" finalist
George Canyon	Country music singer
Kevin Corvais	Singer and "American Idol" finalist
Jeremy Irvine	Actor
Nicole Johnson	Miss America 1999
Nick Jonas	Singer and actor
Bret Michaels	Rock star and "Celebrity Apprentice" winner
Anne Rice	Author
Nat Strand	Doctor and winner of "The Amazing Race"
Sam Talbot	Chef and runner-up on "Top Chef"
Elliot Yamin	Singer and "American Idol" finalist

People with Diabetes Who Do Cool Things

Douglas Cairns	Record-breaking pilot
Robyn Cox	Dolphin trainer
Charlie Kimball	Indy race car driver
David Schultz	Award-winning photographer
Sonia Sotomayor	Supreme Court Justice

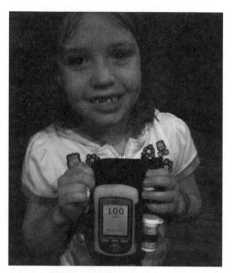

We celebrate a blood sugar reading of 100 by snapping a quick photo.

arbitrary number, but it's a number that is probably within the target range of every person with diabetes. Quinn gets excited every time. Recently, she even had the assistant principal call me at work because a 100 popped up! Similarly, you can celebrate a "no-hitter," which is a day in which all blood sugar checks are within target range. It may seem silly to you, but finding small victories to celebrate can add highlights to the otherwise routine diabetes tasks.

Dealing with Burnout

Just like their caregivers, kids with diabetes are susceptible to burnout. In fact, a large percentage of teens and young adults, particularly those who have been living with type 1 for many years, hit a wall at some point. Suddenly, a once-compliant kid declares, "I don't want to do this anymore!" which, of course, is not an option. But, who can blame them? There is no break from diabetes. A constant schedule of blood sugar checks, injections, carb counting and your well-intended concern can take its toll.

Sometimes burnout is not as blatant, and comes in the form of kids "forgetting" to check their blood sugar, or "forgetting" to bolus for a meal, which makes it harder to recognize. If your child is having erratic readings or an elevated A1c, that could be a sign of burnout. Another sign might be doing all their checks and bolusing behind closed doors.

There is really no way to avoid burnout, but if and when it happens, there are some things you can do to help:

- Be understanding. Let them know that most people struggle with this disease (including you). Acknowledge how hard it is for them.
- Take control. Even if your child has taken on most of his or her own care, burnout is a cry for help. It's time to step back in with reminders and more diligent monitoring.
- Change things up. If they've been taking injections for a long time, maybe it's time to suggest a pump, or vice versa. Talk to a dietitian about new meal choices. Ask for your child's input on what they'd like to change (within reason).
- Never punish. Most kids with diabetes already feel somewhat punished by their diagnosis. You may only push them farther away by getting upset.
- Seek help. If your child is really struggling, it's time to talk to a therapist or counselor, particularly one that understands diabetes issues.

As I will mention in the upcoming chapter on teen issues, some older kids can also benefit from becoming a role model or mentor to younger children. It gives them an opportunity to be empowered and focus on others. Even advocacy and fundraising efforts can make kids feel more in control. Finally, keep reminding them that although diabetes has changed their lives, there are many things that haven't changed, such as sports, friends, hobbies, college, and opportunities for the future.

ART THERAPY

Lee Ann Thill

What do blood glucose checks, insulin, and carb counting have to do with crayons, glue sticks, and glitter? For families living with diabetes, more than you might expect! When parenting a child with diabetes, being a problem-solver is vital to maintaining your child's health, and solving problems requires creativity. Creative problem solving means looking at a set of circumstances, identifying and analyzing possible responses, and taking action—something people managing dia-

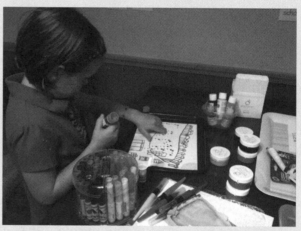

betes do countless times throughout the day, every day.

Families with diabetes have to think outside the box to discover solutions to the challenges of diabetes: whether it's cramming two weeks' worth of supplies into a suitcase for a one-week vacation (just in case!); deciding where to put

Quinn loves creating artwork. Here she is making a piece of art for Diabetes Art Day depicting diabetes camp. She used test strips to write out the words.

the pump in that Halloween costume; responding to people's misinformed comments; or constructively responding to your child if diabetes burnout takes hold. The more often you take opportunities to be creative, the better you'll be able to solve those challenges, and making art strengthens your creative potential.

Many families find themselves struggling with issues beyond balancing basal rates and blood sugar. Diabetes is commonly associated with problems such as sadness and frustration ("I'm tired of diabetes, and I'm tired of trying"); anxiety ("My child is going to the nurse every day with a tummy ache, complaining he wants to go home, but he's not sick!"); family problems ("Managing his diabetes always falls on me!"); and social problems ("Mom,

she said I can't come to her slumber party because I have diabetes!").
When issues like this emerge, diabetes can feel extra burdensome because
in addition to physical health being at stake, so are the aspects of our lives
that contribute to overall quality of life—family and social relationships,
school and work, feelings of self-worth and self-efficacy, and a more general sense of who we are and what diabetes means in our lives.

When faced with these common diabetes difficulties, it can be helpful
to your family, your child, and your child's future physical and emotional
health to consider professional support. Art therapy is a constructive,
engaging, effective, fun, and family-friendly option. Art therapy combines
creative, visual expression with psychotherapy to help people express
and explore thoughts, feelings, and experiences. It is based on the belief
that artistic expression is inherently healing, and reflecting on one's artistic
creations can promote insight and facilitate creative problem solving.

Art therapists are trained to help you identify problems and guide you
in discovering solutions through supportive art-making experiences and
thoughtful discussion. Many of the problems and emotions that come with
diabetes are difficult to talk about, and art making can be a wonderful
tool for expressing feelings and ideas that are hard to put into words.
Children easily and naturally engage in art therapy, but even parents who
might think art therapy "isn't for them" can derive tremendous benefit.
The magic of art therapy is that it requires no talent, only a willingness
to approach problems from a different perspective.

Even without the aid of a therapist, you can reap the rewards of art
therapy. Clear a table, lay out some art materials (drawing supplies, paint,
collage materials, diabetes supplies, anything that feels like it would be
fun), and get to work as a family, just as you'd gather around the table
for dinnertime. Family art-making is a special time to build memories and
connect. Art is an empowering language for children because it's a
language they speak fluently. The younger the child, the less they will have
the exact words to describe how they feel about something, but through

continued on next page

ART THERAPY con't

art, they can express anything. Play with the art materials, tell your story using the art materials just like children do, speak the language of art with them, and most of all, have fun!

When you finish, hang up everyone's art, step back, and look at it together. With a completely open mind, ask your child to tell you about their art. Never assume you know what the objects and narrative behind it are. Allow the meaning to come from your child. Have everyone talk about their art in a similar fashion—"What is your art about?" "Is there a story that goes with it?" Discuss each other's art—what it reminds you of, how it makes you feel, if you recognize something that connects to your experience with diabetes. Create a dialogue with a playful "story time" atmosphere, keep the conversation on their level, and stay attuned to what they might need—reassurance, understanding, affirmation, recognition—and when they're ready to stop talking about it. The length and depth of the conversation will vary depending on children's ages and personalities, but even a short dialogue is an invitation for dialogue in the future.

Remember that some children might not want to talk much at all, and that's okay, too. After all, the point of making the art is to tell a story about diabetes, so the art might say everything that needs to be said. Lastly, diabetes can be an ugly disease, and if the art captures that feeling or experience, then it's still beautiful. Accept it for its honesty and for representing how we all feel about diabetes sometimes.

Lee Ann Thill, MA, ATR-BC, LPC, provides art therapy and counseling to individuals and groups affected by diabetes in her private practice in suburban Philadelphia (www.leeannthill.com). She is Adjunct Professor of Art Therapy at Holy Family University, and she is a national presenter for patient and professional groups about art therapy, mental health, and diabetes. Lee Ann has had type 1 diabetes since 1978, and as an advocate in the Diabetes Online Community, she is founder and facilitator of Diabetes Art Day and the World Diabetes Day Postcard Exchange (www.wddpe.com). She blogs at www.thebuttercompartment.com.

CHAPTER THIRTEEN

Teen Talk

For any parent and adolescent, the teenage years can be a bit challenging. All the usual issues teens face—a growing desire for independence, hormonal changes, peer pressure, struggles with self-image, driving and alcohol—are tricky enough. Now, throw a chronic, potentially life-threatening medical condition into the equation, and these rites of passage can be downright scary. Since my daughter is still young, I have not personally experienced these issues, so I turned to other parents in the diabetes community for some words of wisdom. I also spoke with some type 1 young adults who have successfully navigated these waters, and are now living happy, healthy and independent lives—which means, it can be done!

Moving Toward Independence

At a diabetes camp geared toward parents of adolescents, an experienced counselor stood in front of a group of anxious parents and said something they didn't expect to hear. Instead of telling parents to let go, he told them not to push for complete independence. Although teens want more freedom, most experts agree they still need parental involvement in their diabetes care. He also warned that if you remove yourself totally from their diabetes management, it will be much harder for you to step back in if there is a problem. Instead, he suggested that parents always keep a light hand on the situation. Now, that doesn't mean you should be the dreaded "helicopter parent" who hovers constantly, nagging your kids about checking, monitoring every bite of food they take, and micromanaging their numbers. Parents do need to learn to let go, but it's a delicate balance between giving them independence and keeping a pulse on things.

Parents who have lived through the teen years, as well as most medical care teams, say the same thing: start giving your d-kids age-appropriate responsibilities from the very beginning, building slowly toward independence. How much responsibility you give, and at what age, will depend on the personality and maturity of your child. I know some kids who started doing their own blood sugar checks as early as five or six years old, while others don't feel comfortable about pricking their fingers until much later. However, by middle school, most kids are doing all their own checking, doing injections (or pump site changes), and are no longer relying on the school nurse.

As part of that transition, there should be some discussion about what your expectations are, and what the repercussions will be for not meeting those expectations. Some parents have found that having a written plan, including a schedule for checking, works well, while others use a less structured approach. Some families check meters daily, while others download information once a week and look at trends to see if their teen is on the right track. Again, the method will depend on your child's personality and your own family dynamics. The important thing is to keep communications open and honest.

Your teen wants independence, but with independence comes

responsibilities. So, for instance, your son or daughter may not want to check in with you as often as you'd like, but you still need to make sure your child is safe. Creating a compromise—"if you want to go to the dance, than you have to check in before and after"—can be an effective strategy. Also, working toward a goal may be a good motivator. When her type 1 son wanted to attend a week-long camp in sixth grade, d-mom Melinda Vahradian developed a plan over the months preceding the trip. If her son could demonstrate his ability to handle his care on his own, including pump site changes, then he could go. When the time came to evaluate his progress, she was amazed at how well he did. It also provided a good incentive to improve his math skills!

Like it or not, many kids with type 1 diabetes mature faster than their peers. We try to let them be kids first, but, out of necessity, they are faced with more responsibilities and are forced to grow up faster than other kids their age. This can be an advantage as they move into the teen years. The routines and good habits you've worked hard to establish over the years have undoubtedly become ingrained in your child and will serve him or her well as they move toward independence.

Remember, all teens separate from their parents—it's a natural and healthy part of growing up. And, a certain amount of teenage rebellion is to be expected. However, as Bennet Dunlap, father of two type 1 teenagers and author of *Your Diabetes May Vary* (www.YDMV.net) cautioned, "*While some rebellion against parents is natural, rebellion against diabetes is dangerous! When diabetes care is too parentally driven, it can become a constant point of contention; it can backfire and cause kids to rebel against diabetes as a surrogate for parents.*" It's far better to take a team approach, in which you're working together to ensure children's long-term health by helping them take responsibility for diabetes before the natural separation. That lets them rebel against you, not their diabetes. You are there to offer reminders, support, and guidance, but ultimately, they are responsible for managing their diabetes.

There is no magic formula for raising a teen with diabetes. What works for one kid may not work for another. Some parents have offered incentives for kids to comply with their care, and some have tried taking privileges away—neither has been 100 percent effective. In the end, teens must accept their diabetes and choose to comply on their own—with your support.

TIPS FOR TRANSITIONING TO INDEPENDENCE

- As soon as it's practical, start giving your child age-appropriate responsibilities in his or her care.
- Lay a strong foundation by establishing routines and good habits early on that will become part of your child's life.
- Learn to trust your child. When he or she starts asking for more independence, don't discourage it. Instead, have a "trial period." Let them be responsible for their care for a specified time period, while you stay "hands off" (yes, it's tough to do!), and then evaluate.
- Have your child prove his or her trustworthiness prior to a big event or trip. Having a goal can be a great motivator.
- Foster a good relationship between your child and his or her medical care team. When your kids are young, you attend every appointment with them, which teaches them that check-ups are a priority, but one day, they will be responsible for going on their own. Let them participate in appointments by asking questions and sharing concerns, and giving them some time alone, if appropriate.

continued on next page

TIPS FOR TRANSITIONING TO INDEPENDENCE con't

Your son or daughter should feel comfortable talking with the doctor about anything—including issues they may not feel comfortable talking to you about.

- Help your child develop a strong peer group, either through diabetes camps and conferences, or your local community. Close friends who do not have diabetes should be educated on the basics, so they can help your child if necessary.
- Keep communications open and honest. Your teen should never feel a need to hide information from you, or that there's a risk of punishment for not keeping tight control. Avoid using language such as "good and bad" numbers or "good and bad" food; rather it's just information that can be used to make adjustments.
- Check in daily— but not just to ask about his or her numbers. Inquire about friends, homework, sports and other things before asking about diabetes.
- Pick your battles. While occasionally indulging in junk food is no big deal, manipulating meters or otherwise lying about blood sugar is not acceptable.
- Be prepared to take a few steps backward on the road to independence. If you give your teen more responsibility than he or she can handle, rein things in for a while. Don't dwell on mistakes; simply make adjustments and try again.
- Take the long view. Remind teens that they can do anything they want—go to college, have a career, start a family—but they cannot pursue those dreams unless they take care of their health.
- Don't push for complete independence. Most pediatric endocrinologists agree that teens need some direct parental involvement in diabetes care right up until the time they go to college, and sometimes longer.

Wear It Proudly

There is some debate among teens in the diabetes community about whether it's better to be diagnosed when you are very young, or as an older child or young adult. Kids who are diagnosed as young children do not remember life before diabetes. They don't know any other way of doing things. Young children also tend to be more accepting and embrace the condition. As I've mentioned, Quinn will talk to anyone who is willing to listen about her diabetes. It can be tougher for older kids, who now have to adjust their routines and change their habits. However, no matter when kids are diagnosed, attitudes are likely to change as they get older. That sparkly pink diabetes supply bag that was so cute in elementary school is no longer "cool" in middle or high school. Parents need to recognize and adjust to these changing attitudes.

D-mom and blogger Linda Werts (acurefortyler.blogspot.com), whose son was diagnosed when he was 12 years old, recalls sitting in the endocrinologist's office and listening to the nurse tell her son that this was his disease. Although he would always have the love and support of his family, as well as all the help he needed, the responsibility of caring for his diabetes was ultimately his. It sounded harsh at the time, but after being given "ownership" from the beginning, he became incredibly mature and responsible, and is now an active, healthy teenager who manages his condition well. His mom jokes that he is

> ! Even if your child is diagnosed as a teen, make sure you learn to check blood sugar and give injections. You may never need to do it, but understanding the process is important for you and your child, and may be necessary in an emergency.

much better at remembering to test his blood sugar or have a snack before sports than he is at remembering to clean his room or take out the trash!

A big part of a teen's success is taking ownership, and developing an attitude that diabetes is nothing to be ashamed of or hide from others. For teens already dealing with self-image issues and trying to fit in socially, this can be difficult. Naomi, who was diagnosed with type 1 just two months after her second birthday, is now a college

> ! Your teen is probably away from home a lot, whether at sports practice, working a part-time job, or just hanging out with friends, which makes wearing a medical alert a must! These days, there are more stylish options, such as military-style dog tags and Tiffany-style bracelets, that make wearing one less conspicuous. Having your medical team impress the importance of wearing a medical alert may carry more weight than you making the suggestion.

student and diabetes blogger (Diabeteen.wordpress.com). She remembers starting high school and, not wanting to be different, working hard to keep her diabetes a secret from her classmates. Looking back, she regrets the time and energy she wasted trying to hide her condition instead of enjoying this time in her life. Over the years, she learned that anyone worth having as a friend didn't care whether she had diabetes or not.

Hiding diabetes can not only be dangerous but also may prevent your teen from enjoying all the activities that make these years special, such as dances, sports and parties. If your son or daughter is avoiding social situations or turning down invitations because of diabetes, it's time to step in. At the very least, the people closest to your teen—teachers, coaches, friends—need to know she or he has diabetes. Teens can still do their testing discreetly, if that

! Pay close attention to a teen who suddenly starts doing all bolusing and checking behind closed doors. This secrecy could be a sign that a teen is manipulating the numbers or experiencing burnout. Other signs to look for are sudden weight loss or gain, a drop in grades, or extreme moodiness beyond normal teenage angst. (For more on burnout and support for kids, see chapter 12.)

makes them more comfortable, but remind them that once something is public knowledge, it becomes no big deal. Teens who wear their diabetes proudly not only do a better job complying with their care, they also enjoy being a teenager much more.

Peer Groups

Every parent I spoke with emphasized the importance of having a strong, positive peer group for their teens and young adults. Have you ever noticed that you can tell your child something a thousand times and it doesn't sink in—they either ignore you, or worse, give you the eye roll? Then, someone else—a teacher, coach, friend or even a complete stranger—gives the same advice and it's a revelation! It's enough to make you crazy, but it can work to your advantage. Advice and support from peers who are also dealing with type 1, or just good friends who are willing to learn and be supportive, can go a long way toward helping your teen.

For many families, diabetes camps are a great way to meet other kids with type 1 and find positive young adult role models in counselors. For one young man, who is now attending college, camp experiences were so meaningful that he now mentors younger children and coaches type 1 kids at soccer camp. In fact, being an advocate and helping others has made him feel more empowered with his own diabetes.

But camp is not for everyone. Camps never resonated with

Bennet Dunlap's son. It wasn't until they attended the *Children with Diabetes-Friends for Life* conference, held annually, that his son found the support he needed. The conference hosts groups called "Teen Tracks," which are facilitated by teens with diabetes. Hearing from peers who are successfully managing diabetes and leading full lives was a profound experience for him. He also met several lifelong friends at these conferences.

Let's face it: your teen is likely to spend more time with his or her friends than with you. That's why it's so important for teens to have a group of good friends who are educated in the basics, such as the symptoms and treatments of highs and lows, and how to use a glucagon kit. Not only will this give you some peace of mind, it will provide your teen with a much needed support system.

Car Keys, Please?

I don't know about you, but I still remember the excitement of getting my driver's license and the freedom it represented. Teens with diabetes are no different, but there are some special considerations. In some states, you may be required to submit medical documentation before obtaining a license. Teens should be told upfront that even though getting a low or high while driving may not be their fault, they can be held accountable by law. Driving with low blood sugar is much like driving drunk; reactions will be impaired. So, it's his or her responsibility to check blood sugar before getting behind the wheel.

Parents should set some ground rules right from the start:

- Check blood sugar before

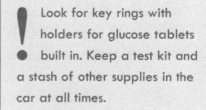

Look for key rings with holders for glucose tablets built in. Keep a test kit and a stash of other supplies in the car at all times.

even starting the engine and treat accordingly.

- Consider setting a higher target range than usual for driving.
- Set time limits on how often to check blood sugar levels when driving. On long trips, it may be every two hours.
- Always have fast-acting carbs in the car, such as a juice box or glucose tabs.
- Pull over immediately if they begin to feel any symptoms, and always pull over to treat symptoms.

Just like kids who speed, text, or drink while driving, make sure your teen knows that acting irresponsibly in regard to diabetes will result in the loss of the car keys.

Alcohol and Drugs

In a perfect world, our kids would always make smart decisions. They would never experiment with drugs or engage in underage drinking. But the world is not perfect. In reality, a large percentage of teens do try drugs or drink alcohol. It can be dangerous for any teen, but it's especially dangerous for those with diabetes. Alcohol lowers blood sugar. It might only take a few drinks at a party to send your teen to the hospital. That's why it's important for parents to talk to their kids, openly and honestly, at an early age, about the risks. And, that conversation should not be a one-time event—it should happen continually.

You don't condone underage drinking, but if your teen chooses to drink, you want her or him to understand the consequences and take steps to be safe. Before taking a drink, a teen should eat a balanced meal or have an appropriate snack. Blood sugar needs to be checked diligently while drinking. And there should always be a trusted friend around just in case. People with diabetes should never, ever drink alone. It may also be a good idea to set an alarm clock for the middle of the night to do a blood sugar check.

When it came time to talk about alcohol, Melinda Vahradian sat down at the computer with her son and researched the risks of drinking with diabetes, including long-term complications. He was so shocked by what he saw that he swore he would never take a drink. Now, being a smart woman, this mom didn't believe he would swear off alcohol forever, but at least he would be educated when he took a drink, and perhaps think twice. Sometimes it's best not to sugarcoat things.

Drugs and diabetes can also be a bad combination. Some teens might think that marijuana is a better option than drinking, since it doesn't lower blood sugar as quickly as alcohol. But, besides being illegal, it impairs your ability to make good decisions, such as remembering to test or saying no to that extra-large carb-laden pizza!

You can also recruit your endocrinologist to help you educate your teen about the ramifications of alcohol and drugs. Sometimes, though, despite all the warnings, teens need to learn lessons on their own. One young woman, who found herself in the hospital following her first college party, has since decided that drinking is not worth all the extra effort, or the risk. Another young college student and athlete, put it best: "I already have to work hard to feel good with diabetes and compete athletically, so why would I do anything to make it harder?"

> ! Is alcohol completely off-limits for people with diabetes? No. The American Diabetes Association says that alcohol in moderation (no more than two drinks a day for an adult) and with food is fine for an adult with diabetes.

Hormones and Sex

Hormones can wreak havoc on blood sugar. Actually, insulin is a hormone, and since all our hormones work together and affect each other, it's no surprise that other hormonal changes may impact the way our bodies process glucose. I joked earlier that it's sometimes hard to tell the difference between the symptoms of lows or highs and typical toddler behavior. Well, the same can be said for typical teenager behavior. Moodiness, forgetfulness, and the desire to sleep until noon are pretty much the norm for teens, but can also indicate that blood sugar is off. Sometimes it can be hard to tell what's really going on.

Just keep in mind that even if your teen is doing his or her best to manage diabetes, hormone fluctuations could cause unexpected highs or lows. Insulin-to-carb ratios may need to be adjusted. Talk to your medical team about how to make adjustments if a teen is experiencing big swings. Some parents say they haven't seen any real effect from hormonal changes, so it may depend on the individual. Of course, whether it affects their diabetes or not, hormones do lead to another important topic: sex.

Having the "sex talk" with your kids can be difficult, but diabetes makes it a bit more complicated. How you approach the topics of abstinence, responsibility and birth control is a very personal decision, but there are practical considerations that need to be addressed. Sex burns carbs, which can lead to lows. It may not sound very romantic, but if teens decide to have sex, they need to think about doing a blood check and having a snack first.

Teen boys who have done some reading or online surfing may be concerned about erectile dysfunction. It used to be a common problem with diabetes, but with today's improved ability to control blood sugar, it's less of an issue. Even if he is waiting to have sex, it might be something he is worried about for the future, so talking to him or having him discuss it with his endocrinologist can help ease his mind. And it provides another good reason to control his diabetes.

For girls, an unplanned pregnancy with diabetes is a special concern. Your daughter should know that most women with diabetes begin taking extra care to keep blood sugar in a tight range when they are planning to have a baby. Without this planning, and proper medical supervision, both the mother's and the baby's health can be jeopardized. Again, it's best not to sugarcoat the facts.

College Days

I had to laugh when Linda Werts told me that when her son announced he wanted to go to college out of state, she immediately began researching real estate there. When her son found out, he said, emphatically, "You are NOT going to college with me!" Realizing he was right, she abandoned her plans to move.

After years of checking on your child in the middle of the night, it can be daunting to send her or him off to college, especially far from home. You don't want diabetes to limit your child in any way, but that doesn't mean you aren't nervous about it! Rest assured, however, that many type 1 teens have left the nest successfully.

Naomi offered a few tips for type 1 college-bound teens:

- Own up to it! Don't be ashamed of your diabetes. Let people know—especially the people you spend the most time with.
- Educate your roommate. If your dorm mate is already a

friend, that's great; but even if she's someone you just met, ask her if she would be willing to learn the basics in case of an emergency. You might be surprised by others' willingness to help.

- Be prepared. Make sure you have extra supplies on hand. An all-night study session is not the time to discover you ran out of lancets!
- Ask a friend to keep a stash of supplies in her dorm room if you spend a lot of time there.
- Don't let yourself get run-down. Between classes, homework, parties, and other college activities, it's easy to lose sleep or skip meals. Try to stick to your routine as much as possible.

Melinda Vahradian, whose son just went off to college, suggested registering with the Disability Resource Center at the university your son or daughter is attending. This gives her son priority during registration for classes (so he can keep a good schedule), and provides some flexibility should he miss classes or tests due to his diabetes.

I was impressed to hear that Melinda's son sends a simple "good morning" text to his mom every day. It takes a little of her worry away and allows them both to get on with their day. If you can't get your son or daughter to agree to "check in" every day, then create a schedule you can both live with. With today's technology, it's easier than ever to keep in touch.

The teen years might seem overwhelming. All parents deal with these tough issues, but as Bennet put it, *"diabetes is a parenting catalyst; it forces us to address these issues sooner rather than later."* Ignoring them won't make them go away, so it's best to deal with them head-on. And remember, there is an entire community of parents who have gone through this, as well as young adults living with type 1 every day. Don't be afraid to reach out to them, either online or in person. They can give you the advice and support you and your teen need.

DIABuLIMIA

Lee Ann Thill

"Diabulimia" is derived from "diabetes" and "bulimia" because it is a type of eating disorder that is specific to people with diabetes who take insulin. Similar to more common eating disorders, like anorexia and bulimia, diabulimia is generally characterized by unhealthy attitudes, perceptions, beliefs and behaviors related to food, body image, and weight. Diabulimia differs because instead of self-starvation or purging through self-induced vomiting, over exercise, or laxative abuse, people with this condition misuse their insulin, skip doses, or take smaller doses than required to maintain target blood sugar levels as a way to reduce or eliminate weight gain or lose weight.

People who practice insulin omission experience the typical symptoms of undiagnosed type 1 diabetes: extreme thirst, frequent urination, lethargy, trouble concentrating, the fruity smelling breath of ketosis, and sudden, unexplained weight loss. Some people with diabulimia maintain a steady weight by overeating without taking sufficient insulin, so weight loss is not always a sign that someone has diabulimia. The primary short-term danger is diabetic ketoacidosis which can result in coma or death. Diabulimia is complicated, insidious, and difficult to diagnose

continued on next page

DIABULIMIA con't

and treat, so the greater concern is long-term complications: increased risk and earlier incidence of diabetic complications, and premature death.

Diabulimia does not refer to a recognized medical condition. It is an informal name that refers to this practice of misusing insulin recognized by endocrinologists and mental health professionals in recent years. The official diagnosis that doctors and mental health service providers assign to it is "Eating Disorder NOS" (Not Otherwise Specified). They might also refer to the "dually diagnosed" patient who has both type 1 diabetes and an eating disorder. Diabulimia is most common in young girls and women with type 1 diabetes, although anyone can develop it. There has been little research to date on effective treatment strategies. Traditional eating disorder treatment approaches are commonly applied when people with diabulimia seek treatment.

Similar to all eating disorders, the heart of the issue with diabulimia is not food, weight, or insulin. The misuse of insulin, focus on weight and body image, and reluctance or fear that insulin will lead to weight gain are seen as symptoms of deeper emotional issues. Diabulimia is very complex in this regard, so early identification and treatment from a mental health professional who works cooperatively with the patient's family and diabetes care team is the key to successful treatment.

While there is no research on preventing diabulimia, based on what is currently known about eating disorders and the psychological impact of diabetes on the individual and the family, there are some steps families can take to minimize the risk:

- Communication between the family and a diabetes treatment team that is supportive and responsive.

- Because the focus on food is thought to increase the risk of eating disorders in people with diabetes, have periodic check-ups with a Registered Dietician for support in promoting healthy food-related attitudes and behaviors.
- Engage in activities that promote positive feelings about diabetes, such as diabetes camp or local support groups.
- Establish a relationship with a mental health provider who is knowledgeable about diabetes for periodic check-ups to explore how the patient and family's feelings and experience with diabetes evolve over time.
- Engage in age-appropriate discussions with your child about their feelings about diabetes, food, and their body, just as you would with other sensitive topics such as sex and substance abuse.
- And most importantly, be a role model for positive body image and good health practices.

Lee Ann Thill, MA, ATR-BC, LPC, provides art therapy and counseling to individuals and groups affected by diabetes in her private practice in suburban Philadelphia. She is Adjunct Professor of Art Therapy at Holy Family University, and she is a national presenter for patient and professional groups about art therapy, mental health, and diabetes. Lee Ann has had type 1 diabetes since 1978, and as an advocate in the Diabetes Online Community, she is founder and facilitator of Diabetes Art Day (see page 214) and the World Diabetes Day Postcard Exchange (www.wddpe.com/). She blogs at www.thebuttercompartment.com/.

CHAPTER FOURTEEN

The Language of Diabetes

Diabetes has its own language. While most of us don't have medical backgrounds, we tend to learn the lingo quickly, and so do our kids. To someone without diabetes, it may sound like you are talking in secret code, as you discuss DKA, A1c, MDIs and CGMs. We have covered many of these common medical terms throughout this book, and I won't attempt to define every one. Instead, I'd like to provide a list of "unofficial" diabetes terms that may soon become part of your vocabulary, as well as offer my perspective on the importance of using positive language.

Diabetes Slang

While we learn a lot of medical jargon associated with caring for a child with diabetes, we also develop our own language, which includes giving dual meaning to common words. People within the diabetes community understand these terms without explanation. Be warned, however, that some of these phrases might cause other people who overhear your conversations to do a double take!

Batman Belt A waist pack (aka a fanny pack) that you wear to carry your diabetes supplies, including CGM receiver, insulin pump, glucose meter, and fast-acting sugar.

Bolus-worthy An item of food that is just so delicious it's
worth getting an extra injection for (e.g., a cupcake).

Cured When you have a string of low or in-range blood sugar
checks, despite giving barely any insulin. It's as if the
pancreas suddenly kicked into gear and started working.
Often said sarcastically "Her blood sugar has been
awesome this week. It's as if she's been cured."

D-Moms and D-Dads Parents of children with diabetes who
function as an artificial pancreas and take on their child's
diabetes as if it's their own.

D-bag The supply bag you carry everywhere with you that
holds various diabetes necessities.

Diabuddy A friend who also has diabetes, perhaps met at
camp or another diabetes-related function.

Diabetes in the Wild Catching a glimpse of someone checking
his or her blood sugar or giving themselves insulin in
public. Also, getting a peek at someone's pump or CGM
in public.

Diabetes Police People who, with little to no working
knowledge of diabetes, question your decisions or care,
as in "Do you think she should really have that piece
of cake?"

Diabeetus (pronounced "di-uh-bee-tuss," like the actor
Wilfred Brimley) You can laugh or roll your eyes every time
you hear him say it.

Diaversary or D-anniversary The anniversary of being
diagnosed with diabetes. It warrants cupcakes, no matter
what your child's dinner blood sugar is. It's a celebration

of *living* with diabetes.

Double Down Two downward arrows on a CGM, indicating that blood sugar is dropping fast.

Flat-lining When the arrow on the CGM monitor points straight across, indicating a stable blood sugar (as opposed to a glucoaster).

Giving the Finger When a parent wants their child to stick out a finger so the parent can get a blood drop for glucose testing.

Glucoaster When blood sugar is up and down, making the CGM monitor look like a rollercoaster with peaks and valleys.

Gusher When you lance the finger and it squirts out huge amounts of blood instead of a tiny drop. Also, when the site bleeds a lot after an injection or site change.

Hoarding Filling your prescriptions as soon as possible, thus creating a stash, just in case there is ever a zombie apocalypse or you lose insurance coverage.

High As in the question, "Are you high?" This always gets a curious look from passers-by when you ask your school-age child, in all seriousness, if he or she is high. You really just want to know if the child feels his or her blood sugar is high, often because the child is acting up in the grocery store.

Mother-birding Holding the straw of a juice box to your child's mouth so that they can drink it while still sleeping, or feeding them glucose tablets or Smarties hand-to-mouth.

No-hitter A period of time, perhaps an entire day, when every blood sugar reading is within range.

Number The blood glucose reading on the meter, as in "What was your lunchtime number?"

Old School Getting away from technology. For instance, taking off the CGM for a period of time, going back to MDI after pumping, or reverting back to a paper logbook instead of downloading data from an insulin pump or glucose meter.

Real People Sick When your child has a cold or other illness that other kids get, not the effects of high or low blood sugar.

Serial Bolus The act of giving multiple small boluses to try and bring a very high blood sugar down. Sometimes done overnight for fear of giving a huge correction and having blood sugar plummet.

Sleep-drinking The ability of a child to suck down a juice box without even waking up.

Stash A bowl or container that holds fast-acting sugar rationed out in 15-carb portions.

SWAG An abbreviation for "scientific wild-ass guess." Often used when looking at a plate of food at a restaurant or a party, and making your best guess as to the number of carbs. You'd be surprised at how many times you are spot on.

Type 3 The loved ones of people with diabetes, who although they personally don't have diabetes, support and care for those who do.

YDMV Abbreviation for "your diabetes may vary." It's the disclaimer given when you describe what works for you, but might work completely differently for someone else.

Zombie Refers to getting up at 2:00 AM to check your child's blood sugar and returning to bed. You might only crack one eye open in hopes you'll actually fall back asleep. "I zombied my way through an extra blood sugar check last night."

Good Numbers vs. Bad Numbers

Because the only way to manage diabetes is through numbers, numbers, and more numbers, it's all too easy to think of these numbers as a grade or a judgment. Trust me, you don't need the judgment, and neither does your child.

Here's the problem. You and your child have an entire lifetime of dealing with diabetes ahead and during that time a number is going to pop up on the screen about 15 gazillion times. If you take that number as a judgment, you and your child risk feeling bad about diabetes ... a lot. See a number, deal with it, and move on.

I caution against calling blood sugar numbers "good" or "bad"

> See a number, deal with it, and move on.

for a couple of reasons. First, you don't want your child to feel that he or she did something wrong. When a high number pops up and Quinn asks me if it's bad, I try my hardest not to use that word. Instead, I might say "it could be better" or explain what we might have done differently to prevent that high number. What I do tell her is that we will give her insulin and get it back down.

The second reason is that as a child gets older and takes on more of the decision-making and control, if she feels that a high number is a judgment, she is more likely to hide it from you. You want your child to be open and honest about diabetes. If a child hides a high blood sugar, then she or he is probably not getting the correct amount of insulin, if any insulin at all, to bring that blood sugar down. Your child may come to fear your reaction.

I'm not trying to make light of high blood sugar, because it definitely needs to be dealt with, but with the long term in mind, what I propose is being conscious of the language you use. You don't want a child to think that having a "bad" blood sugar reading or A1c means that he or she is a "bad" kid.

Accentuate the Positive

There are two words I hear over and over again that really get under my skin— suffers and disease. I read these words in diabetes books, hear them on commercials for diabetes testing supplies, and see them on outreach materials from diabetes organizations wishing to raise money for their causes. It may be only a matter of semantics, but I think the issue is deeper. I believe using these words, and conversely, using the alternates I propose, can shape not only your outlook but also your child's own perceptions.

Let me start right off by saying that my child doesn't "suffer from diabetes." Does she have diabetes? Yes. But suffering implies to me that she is in pain, is prohibited from doing things she would otherwise like to be doing, and is down on her luck. When I am at fundraisers and I hear the emcee ask the attendees to give money for the poor children suffering from diabetes, I get visions in my head of starving children with flies buzzing around them. I think that at any second they are going to parade children across the stage who walk with braces and crutches. I'm in no way implying that I don't have sympathy for children dying of starvation or who have degenerative diseases, such as muscular dystrophy, or that they aren't worthy of fundraising dollars. However, that is not my child, nor is it yours.

My child *lives* with diabetes. See the difference? She has diabetes, but she is living her life. Call it my glass-half-full outlook, but the way you talk about something really shapes attitudes. My child is living a very full life. Yes, it includes dealing with diabetes, something she will have to do every day of her life, but it doesn't hold her back. In fact, she has told me several times she wouldn't want to not have diabetes because it has enabled her to do some pretty cool things and meet some great people. She says she has the "special" kind of diabetes, because she's been in the newspaper, on the radio, and led school assemblies to raise awareness and money. Of course, I would rather she not have diabetes, but in her mind she has reconciled it and is making lemonade from lemons.

Does she have to check blood sugar before dance, ice skating, and swim lessons? Yes. But diabetes doesn't keep her from doing those activities. Do I have to attend parties with her so she can have insulin for the birthday cake? Yes. But she gets to go to parties and have fun. In fact, there are some families I trust enough to let her be at their house without me. As far as I see it, my daughter is not only living with diabetes, but thrives despite it. Using the term "suffers" evokes pity, something that my daughter does not need.

When we were in the hospital at diagnosis, I clearly remember the CDE using the term "medical condition" when describing diabetes. It wasn't until after discharge, when I began reading and researching, that I heard diabetes called a disease.

I don't like the word disease because it has the negative

connotation of being degenerative. Of course, I realize that diabetes is an autoimmune disease or disorder. But again, it's all in the outlook. For me, disease implies that the child will be sickly. The reality is your child can be a healthy child even though her pancreas is broken, which is why I prefer the term "medical condition." She has a medical condition that has to be monitored and attended to, but is healthy in all other ways.

When I was in college, my minor was Women's Studies, and in several classes, we read about and discussed the impacts of positive and negative language. I think it's important to choose empowering language to have a positive outcome, not only on how others perceive you (or your child), but also to help shape your own outlook, and that of your child. In other words, a positive attitude goes a long way!

CHAPTER FIFTEEN

Getting Involved

As you will find, there are lots of opportunities to get involved in advocacy and fundraising groups in the diabetes community; but deciding whether or not to participate in these groups or how much involvement is right for you is a very personal decision. Thanks to the efforts of families just like yours and mine, diabetes awareness and research funds have increased tremendously over the last decade and continue to grow. Getting involved will not only introduce you to other families who share your concerns and experiences, but also help you and your child feel more empowered and in control. However, before signing up, it's a good idea to research all the options, including the background of the organizations you are considering, so you can find the best fit for you and your family.

Advocacy

For me, advocacy takes on two meanings when it comes to diabetes. First, as parents, we advocate for our children, whether it's making sure a 504 plan meets our child's needs at school, or helping to push diabetes-related legislation, such as the *Care of*

Students with Diabetes Act in Illinois, into law. These are acts we do on behalf of our children to better their lives. The second advocacy role involves educating and spreading the word. This might be done through interviews with local media about the lives of children with diabetes, giving a talk at a PTA meeting or teacher in-service about the signs and symptoms of diabetes to help people identify children exhibiting early symptoms, or meeting with your congressional representative through programs such as the JDRF's *Promise to Remember Me* campaign.

Advocacy can help your child directly by making sure he or she is safe at school, or can be for the greater good by encouraging politicians to continue federal spending on research and programs benefiting those living with diabetes. Part of advocacy is identifying the key issues and deciding which ones appeal to you personally. JDRF's advocacy site is a good place to start (advocacy.jdrf.org).

Perhaps one of these topics piques your interest:

- Special Diabetes Program (SDP)
- Healthcare Reform
- Artificial Pancreas Project
- Stem Cell Research

When you've identified an area where you might become an advocate, it's time to read up, do some research, and find other people championing the same cause. As Margaret Mead said, "*Never underestimate the power of a small group of committed people to change the world. In fact, it is the only thing that ever has.*"

And advocacy isn't just for grown-ups. Children can be very powerful advocates, too, both effecting change and educating. I joke that Quinn is "loud and proud" about her medical condition.

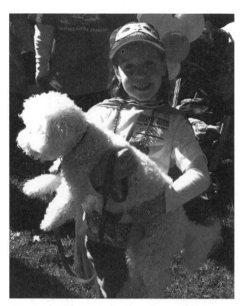

At our local ADA fundraising walk, Quinn took the leash of her friend's dog as we walked the course.

She never passes up an opportunity to tell people about her diabetes. I often recall the time when she was about four and we were in the cafe at the library. She finished eating the snack we had brought and went over to talk with an elderly couple at another table. When her brother finished his snack, and we were ready to return to the children's section, I went over to the threesome. The octogenarian told me that he and Quinn were "talking diabetes," as he was type 2. He and Quinn had been conversing about checking blood sugar!

During a recent trip to the endocrinologist, she taught not one, but two people with diabetes about the insulin pump. The first was a child of about ten who takes five injections a day. Quinn showed her our supply bag and her insulin pump, and then tested her blood sugar. We demonstrated how easy it was to give Quinn insulin for her clementine snack with the pump. The girl and her mother were amazed. When we stopped to dine on our return trip home, we learned that our waitress was recently diagnosed with LADA (latent autoimmune diabetes in adults), and had been having wild blood sugar swings. Quinn once again demonstrated her insulin pump, and the young woman said she was going to talk with her endocrinologist about her options.

Children naturally become advocates because they don't sugarcoat it. They tell it like it is, and are willing to share what they know and feel with others. If your child is ready to get involved, he or she can start as simply as a show-and-tell at school, reading a book about diabetes to classmates and showing the children some of the supplies needed for daily diabetes care. For children who really want to take advocacy to the next step, JDRF facilitates a *Children's Congress on Capitol Hill* every other year where children meet with members of Congress to tell them about life with diabetes and urge the continued funding of diabetes research.

Fundraising

Fundraising is often done through walks, rides, and gala events. Of course awareness is elevated through these events, but the goal is to raise a substantial amount of pooled money, usually for a designated entity, such as one of the major diabetes organizations—the American Diabetes Association (ADA) or the JDRF—or for a specific group conducting cure-based research.

Both the ADA and JDRF walks are family events that take place across the country and are put on by the local chapters of each organization. The walks are typically one to three miles in length. You can raise money online before the walk by e-mailing friends and family and asking for donations. You can also set up an online donation page including your family's story and a photo of your child. Signing up as a team is fun, especially if you can come up with a catchy team name, maybe a play on your child's name, and a great logo. Wearing matching t-shirts on the day of the walk shows your solidarity as a team and demonstrates the support of the team members to your child. Because my daughter has a love of superheroes, and because we think she's an awesome hero, our team wears capes each year. People with diabetes participating in the ADA walks can sign up as a "Red Strider," and each will get a red baseball cap which identifies him or her as a person with diabetes.

The good thing with the ADA and JDRF walks is that there is no fundraising minimum. Let's face it, some years you have extra time, energy, and motivation, and you raise a ton of money. Other years, you just don't have it in you, and that's okay. But don't let that keep you from signing up on walk day. I consider these events more than just fundraisers. I see them as a day to celebrate my daughter and show her that we support her. Whether our family wrote a check for fifty dollars or we raised a thousand dollars, it's not always about the money we put in the envelope.

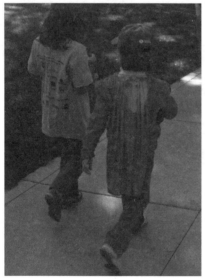

At our local ADA fundraising walk, our team wears capes. Quinn and her friend are also wearing their Red Strider hats, which lets other participants know they have diabetes.

Quinn usually pairs off with a friend who also has diabetes and takes off on the walk course. It gives me a chance to walk with the other child's d-mom, and chat about diabetes and how the kids are doing. I remember one year Quinn and her friend kept running ahead and then doubling back, over and over. They covered way more than the mile we had set out to walk. Needless to say, they both had low blood sugar! It's also good for Quinn to see all the other kids and adults wearing red caps and know she's not alone in this. Though I will say, I cry every time I write out our name badges that say "I'm walking for …" I write "Quinn" on the badges that each of her teammates will wear, and on the last one, the one that is for her, I write "myself." Gets me every time!

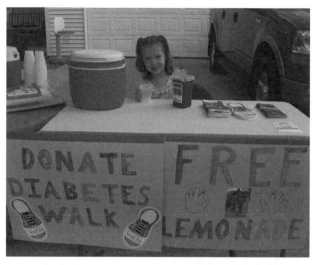

Quinn had a lemonade stand to raise money for the annual walk.

If you are more hardcore, maybe you should consider a bike ride. Annual rides are 30 to 100 miles in length and are offered at a limited number of locations throughout the country. Not only must you get your body in shape—training for a ride like this takes months—but there is also a fundraising minimum to partici-pate of $2,000 or more. The good news is that both JDRF and ADA have team leaders to help you train and reach your fundraising goal.

> ! Some walks will take a percentage of your fund-raising dollars and apply them to your child's diabetes camp fee the following summer. Ask about this option when you sign up.

Fundraising Ideas

You've signed up for a fundraising event, but how do you actually reach that monetary goal you set? Sometimes it's as easy

SHE KISSED A PIG

We were asked if we would consider our daughter to be a candidate for the local American Diabetes Association chapter annual Kiss-a-Pig gala. Why a pig? To celebrate the pigs' role as an early source of insulin. Plus, piglets are cute! We knew it would be a lot of work, but Quinn was pretty enthusiastic about participating. And the good news is that they only ask you once! (Though she could do it again as an adult.)

Our fundraising efforts were far-reaching. I can't count how many e-mails I sent and phone calls I made. In addition, we had a few wonderful people, whom we can't thank

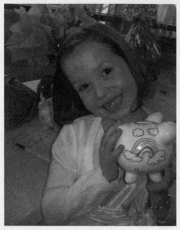

Quinn displaying one of the piggy banks that she painted to be auctioned off at the Kiss-a-Pig gala.

enough, raise funds on our behalf by bringing in sponsorships, advertising, and auction items. Not to mention the cash that poured in from our friends through our online site.

I was undecided if I wanted to involve her school in our fundraising efforts, because I try not to make her seem different because of her diabetes. But I am glad that we did because we found so much support from the students and staff, and I was able to reiterate the signs and symptoms of diabetes in the materials I sent home to families. We had a little friendly competition between the classes to see which could raise the most money. Of course, Quinn's class raised the most because she asked to speak to the class and tell them why she was raising money.

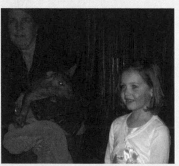

Quinn with Penelope the Pig at the Kiss-a-Pig gala.

We enticed the school by promising that if we raised over $500, their principal would also kiss a pig. During the assembly, which I led, Quinn kept grabbing the microphone from me! She was so comfortable speaking in front of the entire school that I think Oprah may have found her replacement. The kids chanted, "Kiss the pig!" as the principal puckered up.

Her campaign also included talking with media and making several appearances. She was so graceful, smart, and witty. And what amazed me was that she spent a lot of her time talking not about herself, but the others who helped her, such as the classmate who raised $250 by going door-to-door and her principal who agreed to kiss a pig in front of the whole school.

Quinn painted three piggy banks that were auctioned off the night of the gala. I think they brought in close to $100. I liked that she was so interested in finding something she could do to raise money. She also painted a pig for her classmate and one for her friend at school who also has diabetes.

At the gala, each candidate was asked why he or she wanted to kiss the pig. All were personally affected by diabetes, either because they themselves had type 1 or type 2 diabetes or a family member did. Quinn was a doll up on stage with the local news anchors. And she was so comfortable speaking in front of 350 people!

It was a long evening, and she fell asleep on my lap. We had to wake her up at 10:30 for the kissing of Penelope the Pig. She wasn't the top fundraiser, but our team raised $9,000, far exceeding our goal.

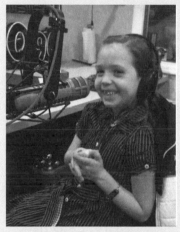

Quinn is being interviewed on the radio about diabetes and her Kiss-a-Pig campaign.

When I asked Quinn what she liked about the entire campaign and gala, she said, "I loved everything about it. Every single thing."

I think she will be a great diabetes advocate in her lifetime, and seeing her interact with children and adults over those four months during the campaign I am confident that she can attain her career goal of being a singer/dancer/actress (and also scientist and artist), unless she changes her mind between now and college. She was so poised and composed, and we couldn't be more proud of her!

Let me just tell you one thing I learned about Quinn: She can work a room!

as setting up a webpage through the organization and e-mailing everyone you know. They are especially apt to donate big if it has only been a short time since diagnosis. But there are lots of other ways to raise money that can include your entire family, especially the kids.

- Set up a lemonade stand. Have your child draw a big sign that says "Free Lemonade" and "Donate for Diabetes." The free lemonade will draw people in and they can give as little or as much as they want. We held our lemonade stand during a neighborhood-wide garage sale, which brought traffic to our street.
- Dimes for diabetes. Have a fundraiser at your office or school encouraging people to fill plastic soda bottles with dimes. A 20-ounce soda bottle holds about $100 in dimes. Have a competition to see which office department or class raises the most.
- Caps for a cure. Kids and teachers can't normally wear hats during the school day. Have kids pay a dollar each for the privilege of wearing a hat on the designated day; teachers can pay five dollars.
- Auction it off. Ask everyone you know to donate a product or service to the live or silent auction at the event. Bundle items to make a bigger package such as a hotel stay, tickets to a sporting event or concert, and a gift certificate to a restaurant.

No Pressure

As I said, sometimes I have it in me to get involved and raise lots of money, and sometimes I show up with a minor contribution.

And there's no shame in that. You have to do what you can when you can—sometimes it's a lot and sometimes it's a little. Parents occasionally tell me they have too much going on to raise funds, and I tell them to come meet us at the walk anyway. It's a great opportunity to see friends and chat with reps from the diabetes companies who are there showing off their wares ... and sometimes giving free samples!

If you don't have the resources to make a large donation or don't have the time ahead of the event, consider offering your time during the event. You can volunteer to help sign people in, hand out t-shirts, or put out lunch. These groups are also looking for volunteers on a longer-term basis to serve on planning committees.

I know there are some people who are more in favor of one organization over another. Some parents are focused solely on a cure, so they only support JDRF to the exclusion of the ADA, which some see as catering more toward type 2 diabetes. But I feel it doesn't have to be "all or nothing" when focusing your money and your support. For instance, the ADA has a chapter that is active in our town, holds the annual walk, and runs the diabetes camp that my child will attend. So even if, as a whole, ADA tends to use a lot of their resources on those with type 2 diabetes, locally we see a benefit from their programs. On the other hand, there is not a local JDRF chapter, but because they have a statewide mentoring program, I chose to be trained as a mentor to help local families who need guidance or have questions. Look at each organization, including those other than the ADA and JDRF, to see what they have to offer your family and your community.

RIDE of THE CENTURY

Tiburon Erickson

My son, Ethan, was diagnosed with type 1 diabetes in 2004 at the age of four. The diagnosis was heartbreaking. As a parent, you try to do everything you can to help your kids and keep them safe. When the doctor said, "He has diabetes," my heart ripped in two. They admitted him to the hospital, and I spent the first couple of days going through the motions—I completely shut down. On the third day, as I sat in the Forever Young playroom at Primary Children's Medical Center, I had an epiphany. It could be worse—so much worse. There were kids in that hospital who would never walk again. Kids who may only live another year, or month, or day. There were kids with cancer and leukemia and congenital heart conditions. Ethan only had diabetes. We would learn how to manage it, and he would be able to walk and run and play sports and get married and have kids and lead a pretty normal life.

I changed that day. I suddenly had a cause to fight for. I went home and started doing research. I read everything I could get my hands on. We enrolled in studies. We taught Ethan about his disease. And most importantly, we found an organization to put our time and energy into. The Juvenile Diabetes Research Foundation (JDRF) is our charity of choice, as we feel they are raising the money, doing the research, and finding the breakthroughs that will lead to a cure. Additionally, they are focused on finding a cure for type 1 (juvenile) diabetes versus education or type 2.

In 2004, I began by raising money and participating in the Walk to Cure Diabetes, but decided I could do so much more than raise $1,000 every year. I searched online and discovered a destination charity bike ride through the JDRF—The Ride to Cure Diabetes. But it was going to be a challenge. The ride was 100 miles, which is called a "century ride." First, I hadn't ridden a bike in over 20 years. I didn't even OWN a bike. I don't think I had ever ridden a mile on a bike—much less 100 miles! And, how was I going to raise the $4,000 to participate? Economic times were (and still are) tough!

As it turned out, it didn't take much. I wrote letters and emails to everyone I know, and I made a post or two on my blog about this major endeavor I was taking on. People responded! I managed to raise the money in a little over a month. It still amazes me how many people will support a mom who is trying to do something for her child. I was also humbled. I trained for five months and made my way to Sonoma, California, for my very first ride. It was an experience that I cannot put into words.

There is something so remarkable about being with a group of people who are all fighting for the same thing—people who have all done the work and raised the money to get to that same point—people who speak your same language. I immersed myself in the experience, and even though I was only able to complete 62 miles before injuring my knee, I vowed that I would be back.

The next year I was champing at the bit to get registered again. I signed up to ride 111 miles in Tucson, Arizona. I set a fundraising goal of $6,000 and began the process all over again. The economy had gotten worse. In addition to e-mails, letters, and blog posts, I had to take it a step further. Several people said they couldn't afford to donate money, but had a craft or collectible of some kind they could donate toward the cause. So, I organized an online charity auction through eBay. The event took a few months to organize and execute, but after soliciting donations from friends, I was able to put together a very successful auction. With everything from signed sports memorabilia, hotel stays, crafts, iPods, and artwork, I was able to raise nearly $2,000 from the auction and push my fundraising total to over $5,800. And I was off to Tucson! That ride was one of the highlights of my life. I rode hard, I worked hard, I cried hard, and I crossed the finish line.

I returned to Tucson the following year—not only to ride, but as a coach for the program. Every year that I participate, I grow in spirit, confidence, and love for the type 1 diabetes community. I will participate in the

continued on next page

RIDE OF THE CENTURY con't

JDRF Ride to Cure Diabetes for as long as I can ride a bike—and when I can no longer ride, I will be at a rest stop handing out peanut butter sandwiches. The Ride to Cure is magical. If you ever thought raising the money and riding your bike 100 miles was impossible, give it a try— you just might surprise yourself!

Tiburon Erickson is the mother of Ethan, who was diagnosed with type 1 diabetes at the age of 4. She is the coach of the Utah chapter for the Juvenile Diabetes Research Foundation's Ride to Cure Diabetes and serves on the JDRF Board of Directors for the Utah chapter, which seeks to find a cure for diabetes and its complications through the support of research.

CHAPTER SIXTEEN

Looking Toward the Future

The year of 2011 marked the 90th anniversary of the discovery of insulin by Banting and Best. As the first human patients were treated with this new medicine, it was hailed as a miracle cure, because those diagnosed with type 1 diabetes before this monumental innovation were handed a death sentence. While we certainly owe our children's lives to the discovery of insulin, those of us dealing with diabetes in the twenty-first century can say, adamantly, that insulin is not a cure. It keeps our children alive, but it doesn't take diabetes away from them. That being said, I am very optimistic about the future.

There have been many advances in treatments in the past two decades, which make living with diabetes easier and more manageable. Pharmaceutical companies have developed more rapidly acting insulin, which helps to reduce blood sugar spikes. Blood glucose meters are small enough to pop in a pocket or purse and require very little blood applied to test strips. Injections can be given by thin syringes, which hurt less, and by insulin pens, which are convenient and less scary. Kids can even use insulin pumps to receive insulin without multiple injections each day, and they can wear a continuous glucose monitor to alert them when their blood sugar is dropping quickly. Some adults living with diabetes can recount childhoods where their parents had to sharpen syringes by hand. They received NPH and regular insulin that had to be timed perfectly to avoid huge blood sugar swings, and they tested blood sugar only a couple of times a day with large meters that weren't convenient to carry around. Our children have the benefit of newer and better treatments that make diabetes management less of a pain, both literally and figuratively.

Not only do recent advancements make living with diabetes a little easier, they also help people avoid complications in the future, such as kidney disease, blindness, and amputations. In fact, *Diabetes Care*, a publication of the American Diabetes Association, reported *"The rate of leg and foot amputations among U.S. adults aged 40 years and older with diagnosed diabetes declined by 65% between 1996 and 2008, according to a new study by the Centers for Disease Control and Prevention (CDC). Better blood glucose (sugar) control, foot care, and diabetes management, along with a drop in heart disease, likely helped cut the number of amputations, according to CDC researchers."* (http://care.diabetesjournals.org/content/35/2/273.abstract)

At diagnosis, I think we were told people with diabetes live, on average, 10 years less than people without it. I personally chalk up this difference to the fact that people in their 50s, 60s, or 70s living with diabetes have not had a lifetime of modern diabetes treatments like our children have, including fast-acting insulin, and the ability to check blood sugar multiple times a day and actually react to that blood sugar to bring it back into an acceptable range.

I recently read that this generation (not people with diabetes, specifically, but all young kids) may be the first generation in modern history with a life expectancy shorter than their parents, probably because of dietary and exercise factors. However, we, as parents of children with diabetes, are hopefully instilling good eating and exercise habits in our d-kids. I wouldn't doubt they end up being healthier in the long run than their peers, because they are more aware of the foods they consume and the need to stay healthy. That's right, our d-kids may outlive their peers, despite this chronic medical condition.

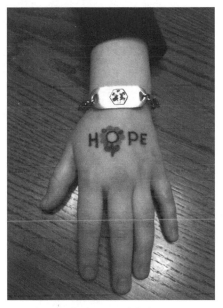

We "hope" for a great life for Quinn, despite diabetes.

Some parents were told at diagnosis that a cure for diabetes is foreseeable within 10 years. For some, that decade has come and gone. There is hope for a cure someday, for there are several lines of research currently being conducted that look promising. This research for a biological cure includes islet cell replacement or regeneration, and reversing the body's autoimmune attack on beta cells. Adding to the optimism are recent studies showing that some people with diabetes still have beta cells and produce some insulin for decades after diagnosis, and that onset may take longer than previously believed.

My personal philosophy is that we should not live for a cure. Of course, I support cure-based research, but I also feel it's important to support research and clinical trials, such as the artificial pancreas project, which can help us manage our children's diabetes to keep them healthy and give them the best possible life they can have with diabetes. After all, don't we want them to be in the best health possible, both mentally and physically, if and when a true biological cure is available?

The future for kids with type 1 diabetes is brighter than it used to be. In fact, it's only getting better and better. With continued advocacy, education, research, and the new developments I hear about almost daily, who knows what the future will bring for our T1 kiddos? I just know it will be great!

Resources

Here are some of the resources mentioned in the book that I find particularly useful. For a complete and up-to-date listing of great resources, including links to various websites, please visit www.KidsFirstDiabetesSecond.com.

Newly Diagnosed

Diabetes Research Institute — Parents Empowering Parents
    www.diabetesresearch.org/pepsquad
JDRF Bag of Hope (includes Rufus the Bear with Diabetes)
    www.jdrf.org/index.cfm?page_id=110888

Books

Borushek, Allan. *The CalorieKing,*
    Family Health Publications, 2011
Betschart, Jean. *Diabetes Care for Babies, Toddlers,
    and Preschoolers,* Wiley, 1998
Chase, H. Peter. *A First Book for Understanding Diabetes,*
    Hilton Publishing, 2008
Higginson, Shelia Sweeny. *Mickey Mouse Clubhouse:
    Coco and Goofy's Goofy Day,* Disney Press, 2007

Walsh, John. *Pumping Insulin,* Torrey Pines Press, 2006

Scheiner, Gary. *Think Like a Pancreas,*
    Da Capo Lifelong Books, 2012

Scheiner, Gary. *The Ultimate Guide to Accurate Carb Counting,*
    Da Capo Lifelong Books, 2006

McCarthy, Moira and Kushner, Jake. *The Everything Parent's Guide to Children with Juvenile Diabetes,*
    Adams Media, 2007

Chase, H. Peter. *Understanding Diabetes,*
    Children's Diabetes Foundation, 2006

Chase, H. Peter. *Understanding Insulin Pumps and Continuous Glucose Monitors,* Children's Diabetes Foundation, 2007

Vieira, Ginger. *Your Diabetes Science Experiment,*
    Living in Progress Publishing, 2011

Organizations

American Diabetes Association (ADA) *www.diabetes.org*

Juvenile Diabetes Research Foundation (JDRF) *www.jdrf.org*

TuDiabetes *www.tudiabetes.org*

Children with Diabetes *www.childrenwithdiabetes.com*

Juvenation (JDRF) *www.juvenation.org*

Diabetes Research Institution *www.diabetesresearch.org*

Blogs

Children with Diabetes

Arden's Day, written by Scott Benner
    www.ardensday.com

Bleeding Finger, written by Tim Brand
    www.bleedingfinger.com

D-Mom Blog, written by Leighann Calentine
  www.d-mom.com
Diabetes DAD Blog, written by Tom Karlya
  www.dlife.com/diabetesdad
Stacey Simms Blog, written by Stacey Simms
  www.blog.wbt.com/stacey
Sweet 2 the Soul, written by Heather Brand
  www.sweet2thesoul.blogspot.com
This is Caleb, written by Lorraine Sisto
  thisiscaleb.wordpress.com

Teens and College Age Kids

The Betes Now
  www.theBetesNOW.com
A Cure for Tyler, written by Linda Werts
  www.acurefortyler.blogspot.com
Diabeteen, written by Naomi
  www.diabeteen.wordpress.com
Pancreas On My Sleeve, written by Naomi
  www.pancreasonmysleeve.com
Your Diabetes May Vary, written by Bennet Dunlap
  www.YDMV.net

Adults with Diabetes

Bitter-Sweet, written by Karen Graffeo
  www.bittersweetdiabetes.com
The Butter Compartment, written by Lee Ann Thill
  www.thebuttercompartment.com
C's Life With D, written by Courtney Slater
  www.cslifewithd.blogspot.com

Diabetesaliciousness, written by Kelly Kunik
www.diabetesaliciousness.blogspot.com

Diabetes Mine, edited by Amy Tenderich and Allison Blass
www.diabetesmine.com

Lemonade Life, written by Allison Blass
www.lemonadelife.com

Living in Progress, written by Ginger Vieira
www.living-in-progress.com

Six Until Me, written by Kerri Morrone Sparling
www.sixuntilme.com

Food

Gluten Free Eating, written by Jennie Rallison
www.eatglutenfreelikeme.blogspot.com

Just a Bunch of Momsense, written by Becka Siegel
www.justabunchofmomsense.com

Diabetes at School

American Diabetes Association "Safe at School"
www.diabetes.org/living-with-diabetes/parents-and-kids/ diabetes-care-at-school

JDRF "Type 1 Diabetes in School" (including their School Advisory Kit)
www.jdrf.org/index.cfm?page_id=103439

Children With Diabetes (includes numerous sample 504 plans)
www.childrenwithdiabetes.com/504

The American Diabetes Association listing of policies by state
*www.diabetes.org/living-with-diabetes/parents-and-kids/
diabetes-care-at-school/legal-protections/
state-laws-and-policies.html*

The Care of Students with Diabetes Act in Illinois
www.thecareact.com

Babysitting

SafeSittings (diabetes babysitting service)
www.safesittings.com

CWD's Family Support Network
www.childrenwithdiabetes.com/fsn

Travel

Disney With Diabetes
www.disneywithdiabetes.com

TSA Guidelines for Air Travel
www.tsa.gov/travelers/airtravel/specialneeds/index.shtm and
*www.tsa.gov/travelers/airtravel/specialneeds/
editorial_1374.shtm#3*

Sharps Collection

Environmental Protection Agency
www.epa.gov/osw/nonhaz/industrial/medical/disposal.htm

Coalition for Safe Community Needle Disposal
www.safeneedledisposal.org

U.S. Food and Drug Administration
*www.fda.gov/MedicalDevices/ProductsandMedical
Procedures/HomeHealthandConsumer/
ConsumerProducts/Sharps/ucm20025647.htm*

Fundraising

ADA Step Out Walk
www.stepout.diabetes.org

ADA Tour de Cure
www.tour.diabetes.org

JDRF Walk to Cure Diabetes
www.walk.jdrf.org

JDRF Ride to Cure Diabetes
www2.jdrf.org/site/PageServer?pagename=ride_homepage

Fun with Diabetes

Diabetes Art Day
www.diabetesartday.com

You Can Do This Project
www.youcandothisproject.com

World Diabetes Day Postcard Exchange
www.wddpe.com

Camps

ADA Camps
www.diabetes.org/living-with-diabetes/parents-and-kids/ada-camps

Diabetes Education and Camping Association
www.diabetescamps.org

Sports and Adventure

Connected in Motion
www.connectedinmotion.ca

Insulindependence
: *www.insulindependence.org*

Team Type 1
: *www.teamtype1.org*

Advocacy

JDRF Advocacy
: *www.advocacy.jdrf.org*

Diabetes Advocates
: *www.diabetesadvocates.org*

Conferences

Children with Diabetes
: *www.childrenwithdiabetes.com/activities*

Other Online Resources

Caring Bridge
: *www.caringbridge.org*

The USDA National Nutrient Database
: *www.nal.usda.gov/fnic/foodcomp/search*

Pediatric Care Online (list of the carb content of some medications)
: *www.pediatriccareonline.org/pco/ub/view/ Pediatric-Druglookup/153888/0/ carbohydrate_content_of_medications*

Studies and Trials

Joslin 50-Year Medalist Study

www.joslin.org/50_year_medalist_study.html

TrialNet

www.diabetestrialnet.org

Products

Frio Cooling Wallet (keeps insulin cool)

www.frioinsulincoolingcase.com

Medical Alert Temporary Tattoos from SafetyTat
(can customize TatBuilder Basic with phone number
and medical condition)

www.store.safetytat.com

Diabetic Passenger and Driver Car Window Decals
from D.A.D. Innovations

www.dadinnovations.com/products.html

Medical Alert Labels from Name Bubbles
(laminated and waterproof)

www.namebubbles.com/labeldesigns/WPALERT.html

Engraved Medical Alert Bracelets from Lauren's Hope

www.laurenshope.com

iPhone Apps

The CalorieKing

Diabetes Coaching Services

Integrated Diabetes

www.integrateddiabetes.com

Carb Factors of Common Foods
Calculated using the USDA National Nutrient Database
www.nal.usda.gov/fnic/foodcomp/search/

	Carb Factor
Breads	
Bagels	
cinnamon raison	0.552
plain, includes onion, poppy, sesame	0.534
wheat	0.489
Biscuits, plain or buttermilk	0.446
Bread	
French, includes sourdough	0.564
raisin	0.523
white	0.491
whole wheat	0.495
Bun, includes hamburger and hot dog	0.520
Corn bread	0.435
Croissant, butter	0.458
English muffin	0.460
Roll, dinner	0.520
Taco shell	0.627
Tortllla	0.493
Candy	
Caramel	0.770
Chocolate covered raisins	0.684
Chocolate, milk	0.594
Chocolate, semi-sweet	0.639
Fudge	0.764
Jellybeans	0.936
M&M's	0.712
Skittles	0.908
Desserts & Sweets	
Cake	
angelfood, commercially prepared	0.578
cupcakes with frosting	0.672
chocolate, commercially prepared with chocolate frosting	0.528
yellow, commercially prepared with chocolate frosting	0.554

Carb Factors of Common Foods

Calculated using the USDA National Nutrient Database
www.nal.usda.gov/fnic/foodcomp/search/

	Carb Factor
Desserts & Sweets	
Doughnut	
cake, chocolate, sugared or glazed	0.574
cake, plain, chocolate-coated or frosted	0.513
cake, plain, sugared or glazed	0.508
cream filling	0.300
jelly filling	0.390
glazed	0.506
hole, glazed	0.506
honeybun	0.506
Frozen yogurt	
chocolate	0.216
flavors other than chocolate	0.216
vanilla	0.242
Ice cream	
chocolate	0.282
vanilla	0.236
Muffin	
blueberry, commercially prepared	0.495
blueberry, from recipe	0.407
Pie	
apple, commercially prepared	0.340
cherry, commercially prepared	0.398
cherry, from recipe	0.385
pumpkin, commercially prepared	0.348
pumpkin, from recipe	0.264
Pudding	
chocolate ready-to-eat	0.230
vanilla ready-to-eat	0.226
Sherbet, orange	0.304
Sponge cake, commercially prepared	0.611
Fruit	
Apples, raw with skin	0.138
Applesauce, sweetened	0.199
Applesauce, unsweetened	0.113

Carb Factors of Common Foods

Calculated using the USDA National Nutrient Database
www.nal.usda.gov/fnic/foodcomp/search/

	Carb Factor
Fruit	
Avocado	0.085
Bananas	0.228
Blackberries	0.096
Blueberries	0.145
Cantaloupe	0.082
Cherries	0.160
Clementines	0.120
Grapes	0.172
Honeydew	0.091
Kiwi	0.147
Mango	0.150
Oranges	0.118
Peaches	0.095
Pears	0.155
Pineapple	0.131
Plums	0.114
Raisins	0.792
Raspberries	0.119
Strawberries	0.077
Tangerines and mandarin oranges	0.133
Watermelon	0.076
Pasta and Rice (cooked)	
Egg noodles	0.252
Macaroni	0.309
Spaghetti	0.309
Rice	
brown, medium-grain, cooked	0.235
white, short-grain, cooked	0.287
white, steamed, Chinese restaurant	0.339
Snack Foods	
Chips	
potato chips, plain salted	0.508
potato chips, barbecue	0.528

Carb Factors of Common Foods

Calculated using the USDA National Nutrient Database
www.nal.usda.gov/fnic/foodcomp/search/

	Carb Factor
Snack Foods	
Chips	
tortilla, plain yellow	0.669
Cookies	
chocolate chip from recipe	0.582
chocolate chip, refrigerated dough	0.682
oatmeal	0.664
oatmeal raisin	0.684
sugar	0.679
Crackers	
animal	0.741
cheese	0.594
graham (includes plain, honey, cinnamon)	0.768
saltines (includes oyster, soda, soup)	0.743
Nuts	
almonds, dry-roasted	0.212
cashews, dry-roasted	0.327
peanuts, dry-roasted	0.215
Popcorn	
air popped	0.779
caramel, without nuts	0.791
cheese	0.516
microwave, 94% fat free	0.760
oil popped	0.572
Pretzels	
hard	0.798
soft	0.694
Rice Krispies Treats	0.805
Vegetables	
Asparagus, raw	0.039
Beans	
baked, canned, plain or vegetarian	0.211
green, canned, drained	0.043
green, raw	0.070

Carb Factors of Common Foods
Calculated using the USDA National Nutrient Database
www.nal.usda.gov/fnic/foodcomp/search/

	Carb Factor
Vegetables	
Carrots	
baby, raw	0.082
raw	0.096
Cauliflower, raw	0.050
Celery, raw	0.030
Corn, sweet	0.217
Corn, canned, drained	0.186
Cucumber, raw, peeled	0.022
Lettuce	
green leaf	0.028
iceberg	0.030
Peas	
green, raw	0.145
pods, raw	0.076
Peppers, green, raw	0.046
Pickles	
dill or kosher	0.026
sweet, includes bread and butter	0.212
Potatoes	
baked, flesh	0.216
French fries, frozen, home-prepared, oven-heated	0.277
hash browns, home-prepared	0.351
mashed	0.168
sweet, baked in skin	0.207
Spinach, raw	0.036
Tomato	0.039
Zucchini, summer, raw	0.031
Foods With Multiple Components	
Chicken nuggets, fast food	0.163
Fish sticks	0.212
Macaroni and cheese, restaurant, from kids' menu	0.181
Pizza, 14", cheese	
regular crust	0.333
thick crust	0.332
thin crust	0.312

Kitchen Conversion Chart

Dry Measures

Cups	Tablespoons	Teaspoons
1 cup	16 Tbsp	48 tsp
3/4 cup	12 Tbsp	36 tsp
2/3 cup	10 2/3 Tbsp	32 tsp
1/2 cup	8 Tbsp	24 tsp
1/3 cup	5 1/3 Tbsp	26 tsp
1/4 cup	4 Tbsp	12 tsp
1/8 cup	2 Tbsp	6 tsp
–	1 Tbsp	3 tsp

Liquid Measures

Cups	Pints	Quarts	Gallons	Fluid Ounces
16 cups	8 pt	4 qt	1 gal	128 fl oz
8 cups	4 pt	2 qt	1/2 gal	64 fl oz
4 cups	2 pt	1 qt	1/2 gal	32 fl oz
2 cups	1 pt	1/2 qt	–	16 fl oz
1 cup	1/2 pt	1/4 qt	–	8 fl oz

Acknowledgements

If they say it takes a village to raise a child, just think of how many people it takes to raise a child with diabetes. I would like to express my deepest gratitude to my parents, William and Cynthia, who have not only provided childcare for our young family so that Randy and I could work, but continued to do so even after Quinn's diagnosis with diabetes. I know it's not always easy or straight-forward to care for Quinn, but she benefits so much from the time she spends with them. We couldn't ask for a better support system.

I'd also like to voice my appreciation to the staff at both Quinn's preschool and now elementary school. They truly care about her well-being and have been willing to learn what they need to know to help her be happy and safe at school. It's difficult enough to send any child to school and know she is okay; even more so when your child has a chronic medical condition. We are thankful each and every school day for the staff members who are on our side.

I didn't honestly know how I was going to pull off writing a book on top of working outside the home, juggling our busy family life, and somehow managing to get a few hours of sleep each night. My editor Lynne Johnson saw the potential of this book and gave me the confidence to "put pen to paper." My co-writer Robin Porter took my pages of notes and created a table of contents that gave me the structure and direction I needed to actually accomplish this project. The assurances she gave me as she read each chapter let me know I was on the right track. I couldn't have asked for a better team in Lynne and Robin for my first book project.

I want to thank the many people with diabetes and parents of children with diabetes who so graciously wrote sidebars or were interviewed for the book. Their contributions and personal experiences added much depth, which I think readers will appreciate.

The diabetes online community has provided immeasurable support to me these past four years. I have gained so much optimism from seeing adults with Type 1 living rich and fulfilling lives and dealing with whatever diabetes hands them. Because of them, I know my daughter's own life will be wonderful. The parents I have met online are fierce when it comes to getting what their kids need. I draw strength from their experiences. I had no idea when our daughter was diagnosed I would become an advocate and voice for other families. We are all in this together.

Of course I need to thank my family who allowed me to take the time this winter to write. Randy pushed me out of the house each Sunday, tried to keep the kids out of my office, and found things for them to do and see so I could take the time I needed to write. Randy encouraged me to write this book, and has supported my blogging efforts and travels. He is the husband I was meant to have and the father our kids need.

Lastly, I couldn't have asked for better kids. Quinn is an outgoing creature destined for great things. She's becoming a diabetes advocate in her own right, educating people wherever she goes. But she is also so much more than her diabetes. Rowan is an interesting, multi-dimensional child who continually impresses me with his ability to build, analyze, and deconstruct. It's probably not easy to be the sibling of a child who needs so much of our attention. I try to be the best parent I can for them both, and I appreciate their unconditional love and squeeze-y hugs.

Author Biography

Leighann Calentine

When Leighann Calentine's daughter Quinn was diagnosed with type 1 diabetes in 2008 at the age of three, she began sharing their story on her "mommy blog," eventually launching D-Mom Blog (http://www.d-mom.com) to help other parents of children with diabetes. Leighann says that like others dealing with diabetes, she and her husband count carbs, carry juice boxes, and are always on call. She shares how they manage their daughter's diabetes, first with injections and now with an insulin pump, navigate playing several sports, and tackle sending her to public school, all while making sure that Quinn is a child first and that diabetes is second. Leighann has been quoted in Diabetes Forecast giving tips on Halloween with diabetes, is a visible health blogger and advocate, and is a frequent attendee of diabetes-related social media events.

Leighann holds an MA in anthropology and works for a Big 10 university as a paleoethnobotanist. You can often find her looking through a microscope at carbonized plant remains from archaeological sites. Her research interests include Middle Woodland gardening and plant usage in the Midwestern United States.

Robin Porter

With a background in corporate communications, Robin Porter is a versatile freelance writer, who has written a wide variety of materials. Most notably, she has authored several company history/anniversary books, as well as co-authored books on various medical issues. Robin lives with her husband, Alan, and son, Sean, in Canton, Michigan.